These A
They're

MW01503948

*Did you know that . . .*

...cinnamon may fight infection, reduce cholesterol and support healthy blood sugar levels? — *see page 37*

...cranberries contain compounds that may protect against urinary tract infections, stomach ulcers, kidney stones, heart disease and more? — *see page 52*

...red wine and many other grape products contain resveratrol, a natural substance that may be responsible for increased longevity, decreased heart disease and other health benefits associated with Mediterranean diets? — *see page 61*

...stevia, xylitol and agave syrup are all deliciously natural alternatives to refined sugars and artificial sweeteners? — *see page 101*

...good fats called omega-3 fatty acids may protect the heart, fight arthritis and improve brain function? — *see page 111*

...turmeric, the peppery yellow spice associated with Indian cuisine, may prevent cancer and fight the effects of arthritis? — *see page 147*

# 20
# Essential
# Supplements

## Revised and updated

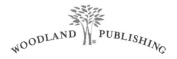
WOODLAND PUBLISHING

For permissions, ordering information, or bulk quantity discounts, contact:
Woodland Publishing, Salt Lake City, Utah
Visit our Web site: www.woodlandpublishing.com
Toll-free number: (800) 777-BOOK

The information in this book is for educational purposes only and is not recommended as a means of diagnosing or treating an illness. All matters concerning physical and mental health should be supervised by a health practitioner knowledgeable in treating that particular condition. Neither the publisher nor the author directly or indirectly dispenses medical advice, nor do they prescribe any remedies or assume any responsibility for those who choose to treat themselves.

Cataloging-in-Publication data is available from the Library of Congress.

ISBN-13: 978-1-58054-173-2

Printed in the United States of America

# Contents

# Essential Supplements: An Introduction

Not so long ago, vitamins, minerals and herbs were not mainstream supplements. Health food stores were not as prevalent as they are today, and people who used dietary supplements were often regarded as "health nuts."

How things have changed. According to the Council for Responsible Nutrition, more than 150 million Americans take some sort of dietary supplement annually, whether that supplement be a multivitamin/mineral formula, a homeopathic remedy or an herbal preparation. This means that close to half of the United States' population uses supplements—to prevent disease, to treat a condition or simply to promote overall health.

Until the early 1990s, supplements were regulated by the Food and Drug Administration (FDA) under the Federal Food, Drug and Cosmetic Act of 1938, which made it difficult for manufacturers to introduce new supplements to the American market.

In 1994, Congress passed the Dietary Supplement Health and

Education Act (DSHEA), which allowed nutritional supplements to be regulated under a different set of rules. DSHEA made manufacturers responsible for the safety of their products and allowed the FDA to remove a product from the market should it prove unsafe.

Under DSHEA, any product with a history of safe use before 1994 can quickly be brought to market. If a product has been used for thousands of years by herbal healers in other cultures, or for decades in other countries where the product is regarded as safe, then that product can be produced and sold in this country without undergoing FDA approval.

## Blessing or Burden?

On one hand, this new freedom in the supplement industry has been a boon to consumers. In 1995, the first year after the new laws took effect, an astounding 20,000 new supplements were introduced to the American marketplace. Each year since, thousands more have been introduced. A simple stroll through the aisles of any health food store clearly demonstrates the widespread effect the new regulations have had on the availability of nutritional supplements.

On the other hand, this new freedom has created an interesting dilemma for consumers, especially for those new to natural health products. It might seem that more products and more choice would benefit the consumer, but things aren't always so simple.

Since the passage of DSHEA, there has been a virtual avalanche of nutritional supplements. And like any industry that presents an opportunity for profit, the natural products industry has attracted some unscrupulous manufacturers, advertisers and marketers who mislead consumers with miraculous health claims and unsubstantiated hype. Whether you're reading the newspaper, watching television or surfing the Internet, you'll find no shortage of products claimed to "fight cancer," "relieve PMS," "provide an amazing energy boost" or "give you the figure you've always wanted."

This is not to say that there aren't nutritional products that deliver what they promise. The problem is that the sheer quantity of new products and their accompanying claims leave many of today's consumers feeling overwhelmed and uncertain of which supplements they should be taking. It seems that only people with the time and resources to wade through the incessant flow of health claims and research could have a reasonable understanding of which supplements provide real and lasting results.

## Which Supplements Should I Take?

It is the current state of the nutritional supplement industry—the influx of new products, the barrage of conflicting "expert" advice and the promises of miraculous results—that sparked the idea for this book. Many people visit their local health food store, see the shelves teeming with new products and wonder, "Which supplement should I take?" With this in mind, the editors at Woodland Publishing compiled a small list of widely available supplements that provide real health benefits and are backed by solid scientific evidence.

The supplements discussed in this book provide wide-ranging benefits and are involved in many vital functions. Of course, there are other legitimate supplements not covered here, and we encourage you to educate yourself about them. But for those who are left bewildered and overwhelmed by the flood of new supplements, hype and contradictory advice, this book is a simple guide to implementing a sound and practical supplement plan.

# Things to Consider when Purchasing and Using Supplements

• An ideal multivitamin/mineral supplement will contain vitamin A, beta-carotene, vitamins C, D, E and K, B-complex vitamins (B6, B12, thiamin, niacin, folic acid, pantothenic acid, biotin and riboflavin), calcium, magnesium, zinc, iodine, selenium, copper, manganese, chromium, molybdenum and possibly iron.

• Most standard multivitamin/mineral products contain enough of each vitamin to meet DRIs (dietary reference intakes, which replaced the recommended daily allowances, or RDAs), while minerals are included in lesser amounts. If your diet does not provide the balance of minerals, you may need to take separate mineral supplements.

• Remember, DRIs provide a starting point, but your individual needs will vary. For instance, pregnant women need at least two times more iron, vitamin D and folic acid than other women. Women who are nursing need more of everything, especially calcium. In fact, if you are nursing, you probably need more nutrients than you did while you were pregnant. Older people also need to consider supplements, as many seniors are deficient in calcium, B vitamins, selenium and vitamin D. Simply stated, your age, sex, dietary habits and lifestyle all have a significant effect on your nutrient needs.

- Generally speaking, you should take your supplements with food. This may help replicate the synergistic action of all the nutrients that naturally occur in food. Moreover, some people experience nausea when taking supplements on an empty stomach. When taking any supplement, read the instructions on the label and follow them carefully.

- Keep your supplements in sealed containers in a cool, dry place. Heat, humidity and exposure to the air can cause some supplements to lose their potency. Keep supplements away from humid places (including bathroom medicine cabinets), and avoid storing them over the stove or in places that are regularly exposed to heat or sunlight.

- Check labels for expiration dates. Supplements may not be effective if used after their expiration date. As a general rule, minerals are quite stable and do not degrade, even when stored for long periods of time. Vitamins are less stable, but can be stored for fairly long periods of time. Herbs vary widely, depending especially on their form (powder, tablet, capsule, liquid and so forth).

- Purchase herbal supplements that have a guaranteed potency and standardized active ingredients. Sometimes, this may require you to do your homework and research different companies and their products. Asking a consultant in a health food store is a good place to start. Additionally, there are many publications that list reputable manufacturers and their line of products.

- Make sure you get the ingredients you're looking for. This can be especially tricky with herbs, as there are numerous genera and species that may share a common name. Additionally, different parts of a plant (roots, leaves, etc.) may have different properties. If the label of an herbal product does not list the genus and species and part of the plant, do not buy that product.

• Follow the label instructions. Do not assume that more is always better.

• If you have allergies, are pregnant or nursing, or are taking other drugs for any condition, consult with a qualified health care provider regarding any supplements you may wish to take.

• If you are considering taking a supplement as therapy for a specific condition, consult with a health care provider. He or she will be able to provide direction and ensure safety while supervising a supplement regimen.

## How to Use This Book

All of the nutritional supplements covered in this book have been studied extensively and are widely regarded as safe and effective, as long as they are used judiciously. For these reasons, they are all excellent choices for preventing disease and improving overall health. Of course, supplements are not intended to replace a healthful, varied diet, only to supplement it—that's why they are called supplements, not replacements.

For a quick overview of any supplement in this book, look for the "Fast Facts" sidebars at the end of each chapter. These include details such as possible benefits, special instructions, safety considerations, side effects and even the best sources for each particular nutrient. The remaining material in each chapter should provide you with the information necessary to decide if a particular supplement is right for you—types of products available, specific benefits, history and so forth.

If you're one of the many people frustrated and overwhelmed by the flood of products, hype and contradictory advice in the nutritional supplements market, this book is for you. Good luck, and good health!

# 1

# Alpha-Lipoic Acid

Alpha-lipoic acid is a naturally occurring substance found throughout the human body and in a variety of foods. While alpha-lipoic acid (ALA) performs several vitamin-like functions, scientists do not classify it as a vitamin because the body can manufacture enough for its own needs. Alpha-lipoic acid is a powerful antioxidant that protects cells against damage caused by free radicals, which can bind to and destroy cellular material in the body, including DNA (for more information on antioxidants, skip ahead to chapter 2). In addition to its own antioxidant activity, ALA helps to recycle other antioxidants, including vitamin C, vitamin E and glutathione, a substance that is essential for intercellular health. While most bioactive compounds are soluble in either water or fat, alpha-lipoic acid is soluble in both, making it especially useful for protecting against free radical damage both inside and outside the body's cells.

Because of its impressive antioxidant properties, researchers have investigated alpha-lipoic acid for its role in preventing and treating conditions believed to be related to oxidative stress, including diabetes, diabetic neuropathy, cataracts and radiation injury. Studies have also shown that ALA may help to protect the brain from damage after a stroke and may even be beneficial for people with AIDS.

Because the body's production of alpha-lipoic acid decreases as we age, some experts believe that a daily ALA supplement may be beneficial for promoting health and preventing disease in middle-aged and elderly adults. Alpha-lipoic acid may also help reverse the decline of mitochondrial energy production that occurs during the normal aging process.

## The "Ideal" Antioxidant?

In an article published in the journal *Free Radical Biology and Medicine*, antioxidant expert Lester Packer, PhD, of the University of California at Berkeley, said, "From a therapeutic viewpoint, few natural antioxidants are ideal. An ideal therapeutic antioxidant would fulfill several criteria. These include absorption from the diet, conversion in cells and tissues into usable form, a variety of antioxidant actions (including interactions with other antioxidants) in both membrane and aqueous phases, and low toxicity." Packer continues, "Alpha-lipoic acid is unique among natural antioxidants in its ability to fulfill all of these requirements, making it a potentially highly effective therapeutic agent in a number of conditions in which oxidative stress has been implicated."

# Food Sources

Organ meats and red meat are the richest food sources of alpha-lipoic acid. Many vegetables—including beets, yams, carrots, potatoes, broccoli and spinach—contain very small amounts of ALA. Because meat is the richest dietary source of alpha-lipoic acid, supplementation may be especially important for vegetarians and vegans.

# Diabetes and Diabetic Neuropathy

Alpha-lipoic acid, in conjunction with other antioxidants such as vitamin E and vitamin C, may be doubly helpful for people with diabetes. By promoting the conversion of sugar into energy in the mitochondria (the energy factory in cells), ALA can help remove excess glucose from the bloodstream and improve insulin function, resulting in decreased insulin resistance. Additionally, researchers have found that patients with diabetic neuropathy—a condition that causes pain, tingling, and numbness in the hands and feet—benefitted significantly from ALA supplementation.

Several research studies support the effectiveness of alpha-lipoic acid in treating diabetic neuropathy. In one double-blind, placebo-controlled trial, scientists assigned 328 participants with type 2 diabetes and diabetic neuropathy to receive either an intravenous infusion of alpha-lipoic acid or a placebo for three weeks. Patients scored their neuropathic symptoms at baseline and throughout the study with the Hamburg Pain Adjective List and the Neuropathy Symptom and Disability Score. The Total Symptom Score was significantly lower in participants taking ALA than in those taking the placebo.

In another study, the SYDNEY trial, 120 participants with

diabetic sensorimotor polyneuropathy were randomly assigned to receive either 600 milligrams of intravenous alpha-lipoic acid or a placebo five days per week for 14 treatments. The ALA group's Total Symptom Score was significantly reduced compared with those receiving the placebo. Finally, a meta-analysis that combined data from the ALADIN I, ALADIN III, SYDNEY and NATHAN II trials showed that patients who used 600 milligrams of intravenous alpha-lipoic acid for three weeks showed a 24.1 percent reduction in Total Symptom Score and a 16 percent reduction in the Neuropathy Impairment Score.

Please note that the studies cited above used intravenous alpha-lipoic acid supplements. The long-term benefits of oral ALA supplements for diabetic neuropathy have not yet been fully established; however, evidence does suggest that 600 milligrams per day of an oral alpha-lipoic acid supplement may help relieve diabetic neuropathy. Responding to the positive news about ALA's role in diabetes and its complications, the American Diabetes Association has stated that alpha-lipoic acid and vitamin E supplements may be helpful in some of the health complications associated with diabetes, including kidney disease, vision problems, heart disease and nerve damage. ALA is a potentially vital supplement for the one in 20 Americans who live with diabetes.

## HIV/AIDS

Recent studies reveal that alpha-lipoic acid's ability to raise glutathione levels can interfere with the replication of HIV, the virus that causes AIDS. In vitro studies have shown that alpha-lipoic inhibits nuclear factor kappa B, which is believed to play an important role in the activation of HIV. T-cell lines infected with HIV and supplemented with alpha-lipoic acid demonstrated a 90 percent reduction in reverse transcriptase activity (reverse transcriptase is an indicator of viral replication).

## Other Health Conditions

Researchers have found evidence that alpha-lipoic acid supplementation may be beneficial in other health conditions, including the following:

- Alcoholic liver disease
- Alzheimer's disease
- Amanita mushroom poisoning
- Cataracts
- Glaucoma
- Heavy metal toxicity
- Radiation injury

## Forms and Usual Dosages

Studies that have found alpha-lipoic acid to be effective in treating diabetic neuropathy and improving blood glucose metabolism have used doses ranging from 100 to 1,200 milligrams per day. Doses of 300 to 600 milligrams per day have been found safe and free of side effects. Studies involving AIDS patients have used 150 milligrams, three times a day.

# Bottom Line

While many antioxidant supplements are available, ALA is unique in its ability to function as both a water- and fat-soluble antioxidant, as well as its role in recycling vitamin C, vitamin E and glutathione. For diabetics, people with other health conditions and even middle-aged and elderly adults who want to maintain optimal health, alpha-lipoic acid is showing great promise.

## ALPHA-LIPOIC ACID FAST FACTS

**Uses and Benefits:** Alpha-lipoic acid is a versatile antioxidant. In addition, ALA may support healthy blood sugar levels, relieve symptoms of diabetic neuropathy, interfere with HIV replication and more.

**Sources:** Red meat and organ meats are the richest dietary sources of alpha-lipoic acid. Some vegetables, including beets, yams, carrots, potatoes, broccoli and spinach, contain small amounts of ALA. ALA supplements are available in health food stores.

**Special Considerations:** Because there are no rich vegetarian sources of alpha-lipoic acid, vegetarians and vegans should consider ALA supplements.

# 2

# Antioxidants

Antioxidants are substances that help protect the human body against damage caused by highly reactive molecules known as free radicals, which accelerate aging and contribute to the development of numerous diseases, including cancer and heart disease, two of the leading killers in the United States.

## Free Radicals

Free radicals are molecules with an odd or unpaired electron that damage DNA in human cells. Normal metabolic processes generate free radicals, but substances such as pesticides, tobacco smoke, radiation and other environmental pollutants can significantly increase free radical production in the body. Free radical damage to human cells can be compared to the oxidation of metal, which results in rust. The human body faces a continual onslaught of free radicals: Dr. Bruce N. Ames, a researcher at the University of California at Berkeley, speculates that cells in the human body are exposed to about 10,000 free radical attacks each day.

## Damaged DNA

Because free radicals have an odd or unpaired electron, they are constantly searching for another electron to create a stable pair. When a free radical takes an electron from a cell in the body, it creates another free radical that is also missing an electron, resulting in a continuous process in which free radicals are regenerated. This process damages cellular DNA and leads to disease and acceleration of the aging process.

The following is a more detailed description of how free radicals damage DNA:

1. Free radicals attack thymine, one of the four nucleotide bases in DNA.

2. As a result, thymidine glycol is formed.

3. The structure of oxidized thymidine changes to a cluster.

4. The cell attempts to repair the damaged part of the DNA by replacing it with new DNA.

5. Numerous DNA repairs lead to more cellular mutations.

6. Cellular mutations can lead to malignant growth.

## Rancid Fats and Cellular Destruction

Free radicals also cause damage by turning fats in the body rancid. This process creates lipofuscin, a brown waste product that leaves age spots on the hands and interferes with synaptic communication in the brain. Lipofuscin deposits are also found in the liver, eyes, heart and other organs. At age 30, the amount of intracellular lipofuscin is about 35 percent; at age 90, lipofuscin levels skyrocket to 78 percent.

Free radicals can also destroy cell membranes, interfering with cells' ability to take in nutrients and expel waste, and rupture cell lysosomes, thus directly entering cells and destroying their contents.

# The Answer Is Antioxidants

A good diet and a healthy lifestyle can help our bodies protect themselves against free radicals and repair free radical damage. Unfortunately, as we age we accumulate a free radical burden that can't always be offset by the antioxidants in our food. Poor nutrition, tobacco use, excessive alcohol consumption and other harmful behaviors accelerate free radical damage and the aging process. One of the best ways to combat aging and avoid disease is to supplement a healthy diet with antioxidants. Antioxidants benefit our bodies in many ways:

- They promote cardiovascular health.

- They control excessive inflammation.

- They maintain healthy cholesterol levels.

- They promote digestive health.

- They boost the immune system.

- They reduce the signs of aging.

## The Nuts and Bolts of Antioxidants

Antioxidants come in many forms—vitamins, minerals, amino acids and enzymes can all have antioxidant capacity. Most plants contain a variety of antioxidant compounds. Some antioxidants work in a lipid (fat) environment and others work in a water environment. Since cells throughout the body contain both water and lipid components, both water-soluble and fat-soluble antioxidants are necessary for optimal health. Antioxidants can help regenerate other antioxidants by recycling electrons among themselves.

## ORAC Value

Antioxidant value is defined as the ability of a compound to reduce the amount of free radicals within the body. In the past 30 years, scientists have developed a procedure to quantify this value. Oxygen radical absorbance capacity, often referred to as the ORAC value, is a measure of the total antioxidant value of foods and other chemical substances. The higher its ORAC value, the more antioxidant value a substance has.

In studies from the U.S. Agricultural Research Service (ARS), scientists found that high-ORAC foods raised the antioxidant power of human blood 10 to 25 percent, prevented loss of long-term memory and learning ability in middle-aged rats, maintained the ability of brain cells in middle-aged rats to respond to a chemical stimulus (a function that normally decreases with age) and protected rats' capillaries against oxygen damage.

"If these findings are borne out in further research, young and middle-aged people may be able to reduce risk of diseases of aging—including senility—simply by adding high-ORAC foods to their diets," said ARS administrator Floyd P. Horn.

# Twelve Important Antioxidants

With so many antioxidants available in health food stores, choosing the right supplements may seem impossible, but it's not. For starters, consider the following 12 antioxidants, which are readily available in health food stores and form the foundation of a strong antioxidant supplement program.

## Vitamin C

Type: Vitamin

Sources: Berries, broccoli, Brussels sprouts, cabbage, citrus fruits, collard greens, cauliflower, guava, kale, melons, spinach, sweet peppers, watercress and turnip greens

## Vitamin E

Type: Vitamin

Sources: Unprocessed vegetable oils, dark-green leafy vegetables, whole grains, nuts and legumes

## Selenium

Type: Mineral

Sources: Meat, especially organ meats and seafood

## Beta-carotene

Type: Carotenoid

Sources: Yellow, orange and green fruits and vegetables such as apricots, carrots, kale, kohlrabi, parsley, spinach and turnip greens

## Lycopene

Type: Carotenoid
Sources: Red and pink fruits such as papaya, pink grapefruit, pink guava, tomatoes and watermelon

## Lutein

Type: Carotenoid
Sources: Egg yolks, corn, broccoli, Brussels sprouts, kale, cabbage, green beans, green peas, spinach and kiwi fruit

## Zeaxanthin

Type: Carotenoid
Sources: Egg yolks, corn, broccoli, Brussels sprouts, kale, cabbage, green beans, green peas, spinach and kiwi fruit

## Proanthocyanidins

Type: Flavonol
Sources: Grape seed extract and Pycnogenol

## Quercetin

Type: Flavonoid
Sources: Green tea, onions and red wine

## Alpha-lipoic acid

Type: Coenzyme
Sources: Red meat, liver and yeast

## N-acetyl cysteine

Type: Amino acid
Sources: Dietary supplements

## Melatonin

Type: Hormone
Sources: Dietary supplements

The value of antioxidants is firmly based in scientific fact. Research on the ability of antioxidants to scavenge free radicals and help prevent disease is too compelling to be ignored. With oxidative stress occurring everywhere in your body, antioxidants provide real support and real solutions to achieving and maintaining optimal health.

---

### ANTIOXIDANT FAST FACTS

**Uses and Benefits:** Because they protect the body from free radical damage, antioxidants may promote cardiovascular health, fight inflammation, help maintain healthy cholesterol levels, promote digestive health, boost the immune system and reduce the signs of aging.

**Sources:** Antioxidants are found in whole, natural foods. Additionally, numerous antioxidant supplements are available in health food stores.

---

# 3

# Carnitine

Carnitine is a protein-like substance that the body synthesizes from two amino acids, methionine and lysine. Carnitine plays a central role in transporting fatty acids to muscle cells, including heart cells, which convert fatty acids to energy. Carnitine also helps maintain healthy levels of cholesterol and triglycerides in the bloodstream and helps prevent unhealthy accumulations of fatty acids in the heart, liver and muscles. The body stores carnitine in skeletal muscles and the heart.

Scientists have conducted a significant amount of clinical research on carnitine's role in human health and have found that carnitine supplementation can help prevent and treat cardiovascular disease, chronic fatigue syndrome, Alzheimer's disease and male infertility.

## Dietary Sources

The body can manufacture all the carnitine it needs if sufficient amounts of lysine and methionine are available. These amino acids are found abundantly in animal products, including beef, pork, chicken, organ meats and dairy products. Additionally, carnitine supplements are available in health food stores.

# Deficiency

Carnitine deficiency is rare, but some studies have found low levels in several groups of patients. According to Michael Murray, ND, author of *The Encyclopedia of Nutritional Supplements*, people with the following conditions may be at risk for carnitine deficiency:

- Dietary deficiency of lysine and methionine, the precursors to carnitine
- Dietary deficiency of any cofactors required for carnitine synthesis, including ascorbic acid, iron, niacin and pyroxidine
- Genetic defects that prevent carnitine synthesis
- Poor intestinal absorption of carnitine
- Kidney or liver dysfunction that interferes with carnitine synthesis
- Defective transport of carnitine
- High metabolic losses of carnitine
- Increased requirements for carnitine due to disease, drugs, metabolic stress or a high-fat diet

Symptoms of carnitine deficiency include muscle weakness, fatigue, chest pain and confusion. If you are at risk for carnitine deficiency and experience any of these symptoms, please consult with your physician.

# Benefits of Carnitine Supplements

## *Cardiovascular Disease*

According to Stephen L. DeFelice, MD, author of *The Carnitine Defense*, "There is compelling scientific evidence that supplemental carnitine offers great cardiovascular benefits. It can not only help prevent heart disease but also helps treat several heart problems, including myocardial ischemia, a lack of oxygen to the heart, and cardiomyopathy, a weak heart, in certain patients. . . . I believe that for a significant number of people, taking carnitine supplements can be a life-saving habit."

Clinical trials and animal studies have confirmed the benefits that carnitine offers for cardiovascular disorders, including myocardial infarction, congestive heart failure, ischemia, arrythmias and peripheral vascular disease.

In a study published in the *American Heart Journal* in 2000, 80 participants were divided into two groups and received two grams of L-carnitine or a placebo every day for three years. At the end of the study, 63 participants were still alive. An analysis of the data revealed that the survival rate was significantly higher in the group that received the carnitine supplement.

Another study, published in the *Postgraduate Medical Journal* in 1996, looked at 101 subjects who were randomly assigned to receive two grams of L-carnitine per day or placebo for 28 days. Researchers found that the subjects taking the carnitine supplement had a significant reduction in the severity of cardiac damage caused by heart attacks. Additionally, the carnitine group experienced significantly fewer cases of angina pectoris (chest pain) and heart failure. The researchers concluded, "It is possible that L-carnitine supplementation in patients with suspected acute myocardial infarction may be protective against cardiac necrosis and complications during the first 28 days."

## Chronic Fatigue Syndrome

Although research is mixed, some studies have found a deficiency of L-carnitine in people with chronic fatigue syndrome. Additionally, researchers have found that carnitine supplementation can help relieve symptoms of chronic fatigue syndrome.

In a study published in the journal *Neuropsychobiology* in 1997, researchers gave three grams of L-carnitine per day to 30 people with chronic fatigue syndrome. After eight weeks of treatment with L-carnitine, participants demonstrated significant clinical improvements in 12 of the 18 parameters measured in the study.

In a more recent study of 90 people with chronic fatigue syndrome that was published in the journal *Psychosomatic Medicine* in 2004, supplementation with acetyl-L-carnitine and propionyl-L-carnitine resulted in significant improvement in both mental fatigue and general fatigue scores among the study's participants. While more research needs to be done on the role of L-carnitine in chronic fatigue syndrome, early results are promising.

## Alzheimer's Disease

Evidence is mounting in favor of carnitine's effectiveness in slowing the rate of neurological deterioration associated with Alzheimer's disease. In a double-blind, placebo-controlled study published in the *Archives of Neurology* in 1992, researchers randomly assigned 30 participants with mild to moderate Alzheimer's disease to receive either three grams of acetyl-L-carnitine per day or a placebo. After six months , subjects in the acetyl-L-carnitine group showed significantly less deterioration in timed cancellation tasks and digital-recall tests. The researchers concluded that, "A subgroup of AD patients aged sixty-five or younger may benefit from treatment with acetyl-L-carnitine."

In another study, published in the journal *Neurology* in 1991, scientists divided 130 people with Alzheimer's disease into two groups: one that received two grams of acetyl-L-carnitine per day and one that received a placebo. Researchers used 14 diagnostic instruments to assess functional and cognitive impairment. While impairment in both groups worsened after one year, the group that received acetyl-L-carnitine showed a slower rate of deterioration in 13 of the 14 diagnostic measurements.

## Male Infertility

Concentrations of L-carnitine can be found in the epididymis and sperm cells of the male reproductive system. Scientists have found that L-carnitine plays a key role in sperm motility and respiration, making adequate carnitine levels essential for male fertility. Clinical research demonstrates that L-carnitine supplementation can benefit men with fertility problems. In a study published in 2005 in the journal *Fertility and Sterility*, researchers gave 30 participants with male infertility two grams of L-carnitine per day for three months. Sperm health was measured at baseline and after carnitine treatment. Results showed that participants who received L-carnitine and had normal mitochondrial function showed a significant increase in sperm motility above baseline levels.

In another study, published in the *Annals of the New York Academy of Sciences* in 2004, researchers wanted to know if carnitine supplementation would reduce infertility among 60 men with low sperm counts, atypical sperm or reduced sperm motility. Participants were given two grams of L-carnitine and one gram of acetyl-L-carnitine or a placebo daily for two months. Men receiving the carnitine supplements demonstrated significantly improved sperm count, motility and form over those receiving placebo.

## Athletic Performance

While athletes and sports enthusiasts have used carnitine supplements to enhance performance, little evidence exists to support the claim that carnitine supplements can enhance energy, stamina or overall athletic performance. Some studies have found, however, that carnitine supplements may help reduce muscle soreness in some athletes.

## Weight Loss

While some people claim that carnitine supplements promote weight loss, little, if any, credible scientific evidence supports this claim.

## Forms and Usual Dosages

L-carnitine and acetyl-L-carnitine supplements are available as tablets, capsules and chewable wafers. Dosages of acetyl-L-carnitine used in studies on cardiovascular disease and Alzheimer's range from 1.5 to three grams per day, with a usual dose of two grams per day. Carnitine supplements may cause nausea and vomiting, especially when taken on an empty stomach, so it's best to take them with meals. If you have heart disease, diabetes, kidney disease, liver disease or any other serious medical condition, be sure to consult with your physician before taking a carnitine supplement.

## CARNITINE FAST FACTS

**Uses and Benefits:** Carnitine supports lipid metabolism and helps maintain healthy triglyceride levels. Carnitine may also benefit people with cardiovascular disease, chronic fatigue syndrome, Alzheimer's disease and male infertility.

**Sources:** The body can produce carnitine from the amino acids lysine and methionine, which are found in animal foods such as beef, pork, chicken, organ meats and dairy products. Carnitine supplements are also available in health food stores.

**Special Considerations:** Carnitine may cause nausea and vomiting, especially on an empty stomach, and should generally be taken with meals. People with serious health conditions, including heart disease, diabetes, kidney disease and liver disease should consult with a physician before taking carnitine supplements.

# 4

# Cinnamon

For thousands of years, people throughout the world have used cinnamon for culinary and medicinal purposes. Native to Ceylon (modern-day Sri Lanka), cinnamon is mentioned in ancient Chinese texts nearly 5,000 years old.

As early as 2000 BC, cinnamon was exported from China to Egypt, where the Egyptians used it as a flavoring, a medicine and even an embalming agent. During the Middle Ages, Arab traders brought cinnamon into Egypt, where it was sold to Italian traders, who kept a tight grip on the cinnamon trade in Europe.

In medieval Europe, most meals were cooked in one pot, including both meat and fruit, and cinnamon helped combine the sweet and savory flavors. When the bubonic plague swept through Europe, sponges soaked in cinnamon and cloves were placed in the rooms of the sick.

Considered rare and precious for centuries, cinnamon has as times been seen as a symbol of power and prestige. Cinnamon was the most sought-after spice during the Age of Discovery and was the reason

## IS IT CINNAMON?

Most "cinnamon" in American grocery stores is in fact cassia (*Cinnamomum cassia*), a close cousin to cinnamon (*Cinnamomum zeylanicum*). Cassia is denser, coarser and less aromatic than cinnamon. Both come from the bark of small evergreen trees, but cassia is not separated from its hard outer bark before drying and does not form perfectly rolled quills like cinnamon. Cassia's flavor is also less delicate than that of true cinnamon.

Cassia has a chemical composition similar to that of cinnamon, and it contains many of the same active ingredients. The United States Pharmacopeia recognizes cassia as cinnamon; therefore, most of the health claims made for cinnamon also apply to cassia.

that many expeditions were launched. Portuguese traders arrived in Ceylon at the start of the sixteenth century and monopolized the trade of Ceylon cinnamon for over 100 years.

By the end of the eighteenth century, cinnamon production had spread to other countries, making the spice more accessible. Today, cinnamon is grown commercially in Java, Sumatra, Brazil, the West Indies, Vietnam, Madagascar and Egypt. The best cinnamon still comes from its birthplace, Sri Lanka (formerly Ceylon), and is known as Ceylon cinnamon or "true cinnamon."

High-quality cinnamon has a light yellowish-brown color and a fragrant smell. To produce the spice, the bark is stripped off the cinnamon tree and then dried. The thin inner bark is then separated from the woody outer bark and rolls into quills as it dries (the Italian word for cinnamon, *canella*, means "little tube"). Today, cinnamon is a key ingredient in treats such as apple pie and sweet rolls, and the scent of cinnamon is familiar in kitchens throughout the United States.

# Medicinal Properties of Cinnamon

Cinnamon has a lot to offer: it is a potent antifungal and antibacterial agent; it helps reduce blood sugar in people with type 2 diabetes; it lowers cholesterol. And this is only a partial list of cinnamon's potential health benefits!

## *Provides Help for Diabetics*

Cinnamon's ability to reduce blood sugar in diabetics was discovered by accident when researchers included apple pie (which is typically spiced with cinnamon) in a study on the effects of common foods on blood sugar. "We expected it to be bad," said Richard Anderson of the U.S. Department of Agriculture's Human Nutrition Research Center, "but it helped."

Diabetes is a disease in which the body is unable to produce or properly use insulin, the hormone that moves glucose (sugar) from the bloodstream to places throughout the body where it can be used as fuel for muscles, the brain and other body systems. In people with type 2 diabetes, the pancreas is unable to produce enough insulin to control blood glucose levels. High blood sugar levels can cause serious damage to the eyes, kidneys and nerves and increase the risk of heart disease and other health problems.

In 2003, Dr. Alam Khan and his colleagues conducted a study using 60 volunteers with type 2 diabetes. The researchers divided the volunteers into two groups of 30. Members of the experimental group received one, three or six grams of cinnamon powder per day for 40 days. Members of the control group received a placebo. After 40 days, blood sugar levels had decreased significantly in the members of all three groups receiving cinnamon. Blood sugar levels did not decrease in the control group.

As it turns out, cinnamon contains a chemical compound that mimics insulin, activating insulin receptors and augmenting insulin's effects in cells. The compound is a water-soluble polyphenol called MHCP, and its effects can also benefit non-diabetics who have blood sugar problems.

## Lowers Cholesterol

Blood triglyceride levels are partially controlled by insulin, which may explain why volunteers in Dr. Khan's study also experienced decreased blood levels of triglycerides and LDL ("bad") cholesterol.

By the end of the 40-day trial, triglyceride levels had decreased in all the volunteers who took cinnamon. The improvement was greatest in the group that took the most cinnamon (six grams). Although cinnamon lowered total cholesterol levels and LDL cholesterol levels, its effects on HDL ("good") cholesterol were insignificant.

Reports from the United States Department of Agriculture (USDA) show that patients who took less than half a teaspoon of cinnamon daily experienced up to a 20 percent decrease in cholesterol and triglyceride levels.

## Reduces High Blood Pressure

The USDA is currently conducting three ongoing studies on the effects of cinnamon on hypertension. Current evidence of cinnamon's antihypertensive properties is mostly anecdotal, so people are anxiously awaiting the results of those tests.

## Kills Bacteria and Fungi

Traditionally used as a preservative for meat, cinnamon has recently been studied for its antimicrobial properties. It has been proven to prevent the growth of most bacteria and fungi, including the stubborn yeast *Candida albicans*.

In 1996, researchers from the Department of Veterans Affairs Medical Center at Brooklyn reported that topical applications of cinnamon oil had improved oral *Candida* infections (thrush) in three out of five patients in a small preliminary trial. In 1999, Israeli researchers reported that cinnamon inhibits the growth of *Helicobacter pylori*, the bacteria that causes ulcers. Cinnamon oil has also been used to treat fungal infections such as athlete's foot.

Because of its powerful antimicrobial properties, scientists are studying cinnamon as a natural food preservative for modern use. In one study, two researchers from Spain's Universidad Miguel Hernández added a few drops of cinnamon oil to 100 milliliters of carrot broth and then refrigerated the broth. In broth not treated with cinnamon oil, the pathogenic bacterium *Bacillus cereus* flourished, whereas cinnamon oil prevented bacterial growth in the broth for up to 60 days.

## Relieves Intestinal Distress

Cinnamon has traditionally been used to relieve gas and cramps in cases of flatulent dyspepsia, intestinal colic, diarrhea and nausea, and it has been approved by German health authorities to treat mild gastrointestinal spasms and appetite loss. The tannin components of cinnamon bark are thought to be responsible for cinnamon's effectiveness as an antidiarrheal agent.

## Prevents Colds and the Flu

The Chinese have used cinnamon as a remedy for influenza and colds for centuries, drinking a cinnamon and ginger tea at the onset of a cold. Chinese people would also swallow a small pinch of powdered cinnamon to warm cold hands and feet, especially at night.

## Prevents Blood Clots

Platelets are cells in the blood that clump together to stop bleeding at the site of trauma or physical injury. But if the platelets clot too much, they can obstruct blood flow and may cause a heart attack or a stroke. This is especially common in the elderly.

Studies show that cinnamaldehyde, a component of cinnamon, has an effect on platelets and may prevent excessive clotting. Because cinnamaldehyde inhibits the release of arachidonic acid—an inflammatory fatty acid in platelet membranes—cinnamon may also have anti-inflammatory properties.

## Boosts Brain Function

In a study on the effects of odor on cognitive processing abilities, participants performed a computerized assessment of cognitive function while exposed to peppermint odor, jasmine odor, cinnamon odor and no odor. Cinnamon was found to improve attention and memory (as was peppermint).

The results of this study have lead researchers to study the effects of cinnamon on cognitive abilities in elderly patients, patients with diseases such as Alzheimer's and people who suffer from test anxiety.

# Dosage

The *German Commission E Monograph* suggests two to four grams (approximately 1/2 to one teaspoon) of cinnamon per day. Cinnamon supplements are available in capsules. Potency varies, so follow the manufacturer's instructions. You can also use cinnamon powder from the grocery store. To prepare a delicious (and healthy) tea, boil 1/2 teaspoon of cinnamon powder for 10 to 15 minutes.

Cinnamon essential oil is very powerful; use no more than a few drops at a time for a period no longer than several days.

Store powdered cinnamon and cinnamon sticks in airtight glass containers in a cool, dry and dark place. Fresh cinnamon has a sweet smell; once that smell is gone, it's probably time to replace your cinnamon.

# Side Effects and Contraindications

Cinnamon has been used in cooking for thousands of years without any discernible harm or side effects. It is not a common allergen, but people with allergies to cinnamon, cassia or Peruvian blossom should avoid it.

Heavy, sustained cinnamon use may cause oral sensitivity, tongue inflammation, skin irritation and increased perspiration. Cinnamon can also irritate the GI tract and increase intestinal activity.

For safety, begin using cinnamon in small amounts, increasing the dose as necessary. Supplemental cinnamon in amounts beyond those normally found in food is not recommended for pregnant or nursing women. As always, consult with a physician before using cinnamon as part of a daily supplement regimen.

# The Bottom Line

The incidence of obesity, diabetes, and pre-diabetic metabolic syndrome is growing at record rates in the United States. Fortunately, cinnamon, with its potential to lower blood sugar levels, may provide a natural solution to these problems. In addition, cinnamon may lower blood cholesterol levels, relieve intestinal distress, prevent colds and flu, prevent dangerous blood clots and boost brain function. Cinnamon may not be the newest, most exciting supplement available, but it may be one of the most useful.

---

## CINNAMON FAST FACTS

**Uses and Benefits:** Cinnamon may help regulate blood sugar, lower cholesterol, reduce blood pressure, fight bacteria and fungi, relieve intestinal distress, prevent colds and influenza, prevent blood clot and boost cognitive function.

**Sources:** Cinnamon is available in the spice section of any grocery store. Additionally, cinnamon supplements are available as capsules, powders and essential oils.

**Special Considerations:** Cinnamon is generally considered safe; however, because continued use may cause irritation, begin with small doses and increase as necessary. Pregnant women and nursing mothers should not take cinnamon in amounts greater than those typically found in food.

# 5

# Coenzyme Q10

Coenzyme Q10 (CoQ10) is found in every cell in the body (CoQ10 is also called *ubiquinone*, because it is ubiquitous). CoQ10 is a fat-soluble, vitamin-like substance that plays an important role in energy production. When we are young, our bodies produce all the CoQ10 we need; however, our ability to produce CoQ10 diminishes as we grow older.

At the cellular level, CoQ10 is most concentrated in the energy-producing mitochondria. CoQ10 is required for the production of adenosine triphosphate (ATP), the primary source of cellular energy. ATP is necessary for muscle movement and protein synthesis; it increases energy and stamina, builds muscles, fights fatigue and preserves muscle fibers.

The highest concentrations of CoQ10 are found in the organs with the highest energy requirements, such as the brain, the liver, the kidneys and especially the heart. The heart contains more CoQ10 than any other organ, which explains why CoQ10 is so frequently associated with heart-health benefits.

In addition to supporting heart health, CoQ10 may be helpful for patients with Parkinson's disease and may stimulate the immune system, boost endurance, support circulation and fight the effects of aging. CoQ10 is also a potent antioxidant.

# Health Benefits of CoQ10

## *CoQ10 for Congestive Heart Failure and More*

Congestive heart failure (CHF), a condition in which the heart cannot pump enough blood to the rest of the body, is associated with increased oxidative stress and decreased CoQ10 levels, leading researchers to believe that CoQ10 supplementation could help patients with the condition. This is not just speculation—CoQ10 has been used in Japan to treat congestive heart failure since 1974, and substantial research supports this application.

In 1994, Italian researchers examined the effects of CoQ10 as a complementary treatment for CHF in more than 2,500 patients. The researchers reported that more than half of the patients experienced improvement of at least three symptoms after 90 days of oral CoQ10 supplementation (50 to 150 milligrams per day).

In 1997, Danish researchers conducted a meta-analysis of eight studies on the effects of CoQ10 in patients with CHF. After reporting that CoQ10 was associated with improvement in five markers of heart health, the researchers concluded that CoQ10 had strong potential as a complementary treatment for CHF.

In 2002, researchers from the University of Toronto conducted a double-blind, placebo-controlled study of a supplement containing carnitine, CoQ10 and taurine in patients with CHF. In the *American Heart Journal*, the researchers reported that the supplement raised levels of all three nutrients in the heart and improved the function of the left ventricle.

The heart-health benefits of CoQ10 go beyond congestive heart failure. In 2003, Australian researchers reviewed eight studies on CoQ10 and hypertension and reported that CoQ10 appeared to decrease blood pressure significantly. Also in 2003, Indian researchers conducted a randomized, double-blind study on the effects of CoQ10 on atherosclerosis. They found that one year of CoQ10 supplementation led to a significant reduction in cardiac events in patients who had previously suffered heart attacks.

## Fighting Parkinson's Disease

CoQ10 shows promise for patients with Parkinson's disease, a progressive neurodegenerative disease that affects the part of the brain responsible for muscle movement and causes tremors in the arms, the legs and the jaw. Although there is no cure for Parkinson's disease, the symptoms are treatable. People with Parkinson's disease have low CoQ10 levels, suggesting a potential therapeutic application for CoQ10 supplements.

In the October 2002 issue of the *Archives of Neurology*, researchers from the University of California at San Diego published a study on the safety and effectiveness of CoQ10 for patients with Parkinson's disease. The researchers randomly assigned patients in the early stages of Parkinson's disease to one of four groups. Every day, members of each group received a dose of CoQ10 (1,200 milligrams, 600 milligrams or 300 milligrams) or a placebo. After 16 months, the ability to perform daily activities (such as walking, bathing and dressing) had declined significantly less in patients receiving CoQ10 than it had in patients receiving a placebo. The researchers reported that the highest doses of CoQ10 were associated with the greatest benefits.

### An Antiaging Antioxidant

As an antioxidant, CoQ10 may protect people from free radicals produced by the body and by environmental toxins. Free radicals have been linked to age-related chronic conditions such as cancer, cardiovascular disease, Alzheimer's disease and diabetes. These conditions are also associated with decreased levels of CoQ10, suggesting that CoQ10 supplements may provide anti-aging benefits.

### A Natural Boost

Because of its importance to cellular energy production, CoQ10 has been reputed to increase energy and endurance. In 2002, Japanese researchers performed a double-blind, placebo-controlled study on the possible endurance-enhancing effects of a supplement containing CoQ10, alpha-lipoic acid, vitamin E and L-carnitine. The test group consisted of 24 middle-aged, sedentary men: half received the CoQ10 supplement for two weeks, and half received a placebo. All performed a cycling endurance test before and after treatment. After two weeks, the men who received the CoQ10 supplement showed significant improvement in their performance on the endurance test. The researchers interpreted this as evidence that CoQ10 supplements increase endurance and stamina.

## Is Coenzyme Q10 Safe?

The October 2007 issue of the *Journal of Toxicological Sciences* included the results of a study on the safety of CoQ10. Researchers fed rats an extremely large daily dose (300, 600 or 1,200 milligrams) of CoQ10 for 13 weeks. By the end of the trial, the researchers had observed no negative side effects.

## Unintended Consequences: Statins and CoQ10

In 2006, naturopathic physician Owen Fonorow alleged in the *Townsend Letter* that "the pharmaceutical giant Merck has known for more than 15 years that statin drugs interfere with CoQ10 biosynthesis, leading to low serum levels, which cause muscles to atrophy."

According to Fonorow, statins interfere with the body's ability to produce CoQ10 and circulate CoQ10 through the bloodstream. In other words, statins, which lower cholesterol levels and supposedly support cardiovascular health, deplete the heart's supply of CoQ10, which is essential for cardiovascular health.

If you are taking statins, discuss your concerns about CoQ10 depletion with your physician. CoQ10 supplements may be the missing piece to your heart-health puzzle.

# The Need for Supplementation

Most of us produce sufficient coenzyme Q10 until we are about 30 years old; after that, production diminishes. It has been shown that as many as 75 percent of people over the age of 50 are deficient in coenzyme Q10.

Without sufficient CoQ10, the heart cannot circulate blood effectively. The people with the most severe CoQ10 deficiencies are those with heart disease. Doctors don't yet know whether CoQ10 deficiency is a cause of heart disease or a result of it. Regardless, coenzyme Q10 is a factor in heart disease, and studies show that as supplementation restores optimal levels of CoQ10, heart function improves, energy production is enhanced, the heart has better ability to contract and antioxidant protection increases. Coenzyme Q10 also helps prevent the buildup of LDL ("bad") cholesterol.

# The Bottom Line

Most young people can produce all the coenzyme Q10 they need; for them, supplements are probably not worth the expense. However, as we age, CoQ10 supplements can help strengthen our hearts and maintain our health. Today, more than 12 million Japanese people take CoQ10 supplements under the direction of their physicians. As Americans continue to learn about the value of CoQ10, the use of CoQ10 will only increase.

---

## COENZYME Q10 FAST FACTS

**Uses and Benefits:** CoQ10 protects and strengthens the heart, helps treat high blood pressure and other cardiovascular diseases, strengthens muscles, stimulates the immune system and fights age-related illness.

**Sources:** CoQ10 supplements are available as capsules, liquids, tablets and sprays. Gel capsules are readily absorbed and easy to swallow.

**Special Considerations:** CoQ10 is best absorbed when taken with fatty foods such as fish or peanut butter. For general health, the recommended dose is 30 to 60 milligrams per day. Higher doses may be recommended for some conditions—consult your physician first. CoQ10 is generally considered safe and free of side effects. In rare cases, stomach upset, diarrhea and nausea have been reported.

# 6

# Cranberries

Cranberries are delicious, whether dried and sweetened or served in cranberry sauce, cranberry juice cocktail or cranberry muffins. But there are other reasons to love cranberries. Current scientific research reveals that the tart red berries are among the most healthful of all berries, and that they have more antioxidant activity than almost any other fruit. As the frequency of cancer, heart disease and other chronic conditions rises throughout the world, researchers are increasingly focusing on cranberries to find new ways to promote good health and prevent disease.

## Cranberry Country

Would you be surprised to learn that the tradition of serving cranberry sauce for Thanksgiving is as old as the holiday itself? Cranberries are indigenous to North America and have grown abundantly in the wild for centuries. Native Americans along the East Coast enjoyed wild cranberries cooked with maple syrup or honey, and they most likely shared this treat with colonists at early Thanksgiving feasts.

Native Americans had other uses for cranberries as well, such as using the berries to make dyes and clean wounds.

In 1816, Henry Hall began cultivating cranberries in Dennis, Massachusetts, and by the 1820s American farmers were exporting cranberries to Europe. In 1840, Hall observed that the berries flourished when sand was fortuitously swept into his bog by strong winds, stifling the growth of shallow weeds and supporting healthy growth of the deep-rooted cranberry bushes. This discovery allowed cranberry production to increase greatly; today, the United States produces 154,000 tons of cranberries each year, the majority of which come from Wisconsin and Massachusetts.

## Cranberries and Urinary Tract Health

Studies suggest that cranberries and cranberry juice may help maintain a healthy urinary tract by preventing the occurrence of urinary tract infections (UTIs). Scientists once believed that a chemical constituent of cranberries called hippuric acid was responsible for preventing UTIs. Early cranberry studies proposed that hippuric acid helped to acidify urine enough to prevent harmful bacteria from causing an infection. However, subsequent studies have failed to prove this theory or demonstrate that hippuric acid in the urinary tract reaches levels sufficient to inhibit bacterial growth.

More recent research suggests a different reason for cranberry's urinary health benefits—cranberry may prevent harmful bacteria from adhering to the urinary tract altogether. A 1998 study suggests that compounds called proanthocyanidins, which are found in cranberries, function similarly to the body's Tamm-Horsfall glycoprotein, which keeps bacteria from adhering to bladder cells.

UTIs are caused by a class of bacteria that includes the *E. coli*, *Proteus* and *Pseudomonas* species. The fimbriae (fringes) that surround these bacteria allow the bacteria to attach to the epithelial cells of the urinary tract and create an infection. However, in an in vitro study published in 1988, researchers at the Alliance City Hospital in Ohio showed that bacterial fimbriae are less likely to stick to the urinary tract after cranberry juice consumption. These results suggest that cranberry is more effective at preventing infections than curing them.

In 1994, researchers at Tufts University conducted a large double-blind, placebo-controlled trial that stands out as one of the most important human trials on cranberry and urinary tract health. The researchers gave 153 elderly women 300 milliliters (10 ounces) of cranberry juice per day for six months and noted the subsequent occurrence of UTIs. The juice-drinking participants experienced fewer UTIs than participants in a placebo group. Additionally, only 15 percent of the juice group had bacteria in their urine, compared to 28 percent of the placebo group.

Cranberry may have other positive effects on the urinary tract. A few preliminary uncontrolled studies have shown that cranberry juice may help reduce the odor of urine and the occasional burning sensation that accompanies urination. Further research is needed to confirm these benefits.

# More Anti-Adherence Benefits

## Ulcers

Most gastric ulcers are caused by *Heliobacter pylori* bacteria, which adhere to the lining of the stomach wall. Results from a 2002 in vitro study published in the journal *Critical Reviews in Food Science and Nutrition* indicate that cranberry juice may help prevent *H. pylori* from adhering to the stomach lining. In this respect, ulcer sufferers may benefit from cranberries in much the same way as those with urinary tract infections.

## Oral Health

In 2002, researchers in Jerusalem noted that a mouthwash containing a unique cranberry compound was able to break up the dental plaque formed by a number of oral bacteria and decrease the salivary level of the *Streptococcus mutans* bacteria that cause tooth decay.

## Genital Herpes

Researchers have studied cranberry's anti-adherence effects on the virus that causes genital herpes. An article published in the *Journal of Science, Food and Agriculture* in 2004 shows that the proanthocyanidin A-1, a compound found in cranberries, may prevent the attachment and penetration of the herpes simplex virus. But like cranberry's effects on the urinary tract, these benefits are only preventive.

# Antioxidants and Free Radicals

Scientists now know that air pollution, cigarette smoke, pesticides, contaminated water and even the food we eat produce harmful free radicals in the body. Free radicals are unstable molecules that cause damage—or oxidation—to healthy cells. This damage can impair the proper functioning of the immune system and lead to infections, chronic disease and cancer. Cranberries are a rich source of antioxidants, which can help eliminate harmful free radicals and protect cellular DNA from the oxidative damage and cell mutations that can lead to cancer.

# Powerful Proanthocyanidins

Scientists use the umbrella term *bioflavonoids* for the many healthful phytochemicals found in fruits and vegetables, herbs, grains, legumes and nuts. Bioflavonoids frequently have antioxidant properties, and some have been found to possess antiviral, anti-inflammatory and antihistamine properties as well. Research suggests that cranberry's exceptional concentration of bioflavonoids may explain cranberry's many health benefits. Proanthocyanidins are just one of the many bioflavonoids that cranberries contain, but research suggests that they are some of the most beneficial.

Proanthocyanidins are potent antioxidants that occur abundantly in blue, red and purple fruits, with cranberries having one of the highest concentrations. In addition to their antioxidant activity, certain proanthocyanidins offer other benefits for a host of health conditions.

The proanthocyanidins found in cranberries help to increase peripheral circulation and thus may help improve vision. In clinical trials of patients with retinal disease, including macular degeneration, patients given proanthocyanidins show significant improvement. Health professionals monitoring the effect of proanthocyanidins on vision have reported that proanthocyanidins also help in the prevention and treatment of glaucoma.

Preliminary animal studies have produced compelling evidence that the antioxidants in cranberries can help keep the mind sharp and free from neurological damage by fighting free radicals in the brain. Proanthocyanidins are among the few antioxidants that cross the blood/brain barrier, thus helping to protect neural tissue. This may explain why these potent chemicals have helped patients with multiple sclerosis and other nerve diseases.

# Cranberries and Cancer

A 2002 study reported that several cranberry compounds—particularly proanthocyanidins—demonstrated toxicity to various cancer cells, including cancers of the breast, prostate, lungs and cervix. This study, in addition to several others, found that whole cranberries fight cancer cells more effectively than cranberry juice. Researchers have concluded that the active compounds in whole cranberries help prevent cancer and decrease tumor growth by halting cell-cycle progression and inducing programmed cell death in cancer cells.

# The Heartening Effects of Cranberry

As scientists continue to study the causes of heart disease, the nation's number-one killer, new research shows that cranberry's antioxidant power may help reduce cholesterol levels and keep hearts healthy.

One in vitro study from the University of Scranton in Pennsylvania suggests that the same cranberry antioxidants that protect against cancer and other chronic diseases may help prevent LDL (bad) cholesterol oxidation. (Oxidized LDL cholesterol is considered a key contributing factor to the hardening of the arteries and heart disease.) Similar studies in animals have concluded that cranberries may also help decrease both LDL and total cholesterol levels.

Further investigation suggests that one particular cranberry antioxidant, pterostilbene, may hold the key to cranberry's heart-health benefits. A study completed by the USDA Agricultural Research Service compared pterostilbene's cholesterol-lowering ability with that of a common lipid-lowering drug, ciprofibrate. The results of the study concluded that pterostilbene was more likely to stimulate cholesterol metabolism than ciprofibrate, thus keeping cholesterol levels healthy and balanced.

Cranberries may also play a part in maintaining blood vessel health, particularly in people with atherosclerosis (hardened arteries). The proanthocyanidins in cranberries help enhance capillary strength and vascular function, which promotes overall heart health and decreases the incidence of varicose veins, leg swelling and retinopathy. A 2005 study from the University of Wisconsin–Madison revealed that when pigs with atherosclerosis were given a daily dose of cranberry powder, their vascular relaxation and blood vessel function improved and became similar to that of healthy pigs. Unhealthy blood vessels can contribute to heart disease, so using cranberries to fight atherosclerosis may help prevent heart attacks and strokes.

## Cranberries and Kidney Stones

The incidence of kidney stones in American adults has risen sharply over the past few decades—primarily in middle-aged white men, but also in women and younger people. While doctors can't definitively explain what causes kidney stones, they hypothesize that genetics, urinary or kidney infections, and even certain foods can cause stones to develop.

Kidney stones are hard, stone-like masses that form when crystallized substances in urine—usually calcium, phosphate and other minerals—build up on the inner walls of the kidney and the ureters connecting the kidney to the bladder. Urine typically contains chemicals that prevent the crystal-like substances from forming, but these chemicals are missing or ineffective in some people. Luckily, cranberries may provide a viable substitute.

Cranberries contain a chemical known as quinic acid, which is not broken down as it passes through the body but instead is excreted mostly unaffected in urine. Clinical studies have shown that quinic acid can make urine just acidic enough to prevent calcium and phosphate ions from combining to form kidney stones, and that quinic acid can reduce the amount of ionized calcium in urine by over 50 percent (a significant amount considering that 75 to 85 percent of kidney stones are composed of calcium salts). Some studies suggest that the acidity of cranberries also plays a minor role in clearing urinary tract infections.

## Safety Issues

Cranberries contain a considerable amount of oxalates. Oxalates are naturally occurring substances that are found in most living things; however, excess oxalates can interfere with calcium absorption and aggravate existing health conditions such as kidney or gallbladder problems.

## How to Add Cranberries to Your Diet

The best way to get the maximum health benefits of cranberry is to mix pure cranberry juice concentrate with a fruit juice of your choice, such as grape juice or apple juice. Cranberry juice concentrate also goes well with club soda (use a little stevia to sweeten the mixture), diet lemon-lime soda and other mixers. Cranberry juice cocktail can be a good choice, but avoid products that contain a lot of added sugar or high-fructose corn syrup.

Another option is to take one of the many cranberry dietary supplements that are now available. Some supplements contain as much as 400 milligrams of whole cranberry juice extract in a single daily capsule.

# Special Instructions

People undergoing chemotherapy and radiation therapy should avoid cranberries and other supplemental antioxidants during treatment, as antioxidants may decrease the effectiveness of the treatment.

# The Bottom Line

The discovery of cranberry's anti-adherence abilities in urinary tract infections has spurred further study into other potential benefits for the prevention of ulcers, oral disease and genital herpes. Cranberry, which may be the most antioxidant-rich common fruit, holds great promise for the fight against cancer, aging and macular degeneration. Cranberry's many antioxidants may also help to maintain a healthy cardiovascular system, thus preventing the onset of heart disease. In addition, cranberries contain phytochemicals such as quinic acid that may help prevent the pain of kidney stones and help maintain a healthy urinary system.

## HEALTH-PROMOTING CONSTITUENTS OF CRANBERRIES

- Anthocyanidins
- Benzoic acid
- Catechins
- Chlorogenic acid
- Ellagic acid
- Epigallocatechin gallate (EGCG)
- Fiber
- Flavonoids
- Folate
- Lignans
- Proanthocyanidins
- Quercetin
- Resveratrol
- Thiamin
- Triterpenoids
- Vitamin A
- Vitamin C

## CRANBERRY FAST FACTS

**Uses and Benefits:** Cranberry inhibits bacterial adhesion and may help prevent urinary tract infections, stomach ulcers, tooth decay and genital herpes. Cranberries also contain powerful antioxidants, which may protect against cancer and promote cardiovascular health. Cranberry may even help prevent kidney stones.

**Sources:** Most cranberry products—sauces, juices and dried fruit—are sweetened with added sugars. Whole cranberries and pure cranberry juice are available, but unsweetened cranberries are extremely tart. Cranberry extracts, available at most health food stores, provide the health benefits of cranberries without excess sugar or astringency.

**Special Considerations:** People undergoing chemotherapy or radiation treatment should avoid cranberry, which may interfere with the treatment.

# 7

# Grape Seed Extract and Resveratrol

You have probably heard about the health benefits of red wine and the studies that link red wine consumption to long life. What you may not know is that grape seed extract provides many of the same benefits. Grape seed extract has amazing antioxidant properties: it protects cells against damage caused by pesticides, food additives and pollution and may be your best defense against the effects of aging.

Recent studies have shown that air pollution, cigarette smoke, pesticides, contaminated water and even the food we eat can produce free radicals, unstable oxygen molecules that damage other cells. Excess free radicals cause oxidation, or oxidative damage, which can impair the proper functioning of the immune system, leading to infections, heart disease and other degenerative diseases. Although not a cure, antioxidants have even been shown to reduce the incidence of cancer.

Grape seed extract fights free radicals and the damage they cause. It can also protect DNA from oxidative damage and cell mutations that can lead to cancer. Until the discovery of grape seed extract, vitamin

C, vitamin E and beta-carotene were considered the best sources of antioxidants. However, these sources are not as powerful as grape seed extract and they are used or excreted shortly after entering the body.

Grape seed extract is more than a powerful antioxidant—it is an antiallergenic, an antihistamine and an anti-inflammatory. It also strengthens blood vessels, improves skin and supports circulation.

Grape seed extract could also play a significant role in weight management. In 2004, researchers from Maastricht University in the Netherlands studied the effects of grape seed extract on energy intake and satiety. The researchers gave 51 people grape seed extract twice a day (30 to 60 minutes before lunch and dinner) for three days. They found that the average calorie intake of those with normal or above-average weight was reduced by four percent, with no noted side effects or changes in satiety.

## The Power of OPCs

Grape seed extract gets its amazing antioxidant power from its high concentration of a group of complex substances known as oligomeric proanthocyanidins (OPCs) or procyanidins. OPCs are found in grape seeds and grape skin; blue, red and purple fruits such as plums, blueberries and cherries; and the bark of the maritime pine tree.

OPCs fight free radicals and oxidative stress in many ways. They also conserve and regenerate vitamins C and E: OPCs work synergistically with vitamin C to regenerate vitamin E (Vitamin E is a powerful free radical scavenger, but it is quickly used up), and these three nutrients then work together to fight off free radicals.

## The Heartening Effects of Grape Seed Extract

Grape seed extract and OPCs may provide several heart-health benefits. The antioxidant effects of OPCs have been shown to inhibit cholesterol oxidation, a key factor leading to hardened arteries and heart disease. In 2000, researchers at Georgetown University Medical Center reported that a combination of OPCs and chromium decreased levels of blood cholesterol, especially LDL ("bad") cholesterol. OPCs have also been shown to prevent the stickiness of blood platelets that can lead to blood clots and strokes. And in 2006, researchers at the University of California, Davis, reported that grape seed extract lowered blood pressure in patients with metabolic syndrome.

Convincing evidence suggests that there is more behind wine's heart-health benefits than alcohol. In 1999, the American Heart Association published a study reporting that purple grape juice improved blood flow and decreased LDL oxidation. The authors concluded that some benefits of red wine and other grape products were independent of alcohol content.

Grape seed extract is good for the nerves, too. OPCs are one of only a few antioxidants that cross the blood-brain barrier and protect neural tissue. This may explain why OPCs help reduce symptoms in patients with nerve diseases such as multiple sclerosis (MS), a syndrome of progressive destruction and hardening of the myelin sheath that surrounds the nerves. It may also explain why patients taking OPC supplements often report improved mental clarity.

Since as early as the 1950s, doctors have observed anti-inflammatory action in OPCs. OPCs inhibit the release and synthesis of inflammatory compounds such as histamine and prostaglandins. OPCs selectively bind to the connective tissue of joints, preventing swelling, promoting healing and decreasing pain. OPCs also inhibit the enzyme responsible for producing histamine and the enzyme that facilitates the release of histamine into the body.

The antihistamine activity of OPCs also may benefit people with allergies and people with ulcers. OPCs have the ability to strengthen the cell membranes of basophils and mast cells, both of which contain allergy-causing chemicals. By strengthening these cell membranes, OPCs inhibit the release of allergy-causing chemicals, preventing overreaction or hypersensitivity to allergens. Stress-related ulcers are linked to excessive secretion of histamine in the stomach lining. OPCs help heal ulcers by reducing histamine secretion and by binding to and protecting connective tissue in mucous membranes.

## The Wonders of Antiaging OPCs

OPCs combat many of the negative effects of the aging process, partly through their ability to enhance immune resistance. Strong immune systems contribute to capillary strength, increase peripheral circulation, reduce skin aging and support skin elasticity. OPCs are some of the most potent immune-enhancing nutrients known: they remain in the body for three days; they are 20 times stronger than vitamin C and 50 times stronger than vitamin E; they are highly bioavailable; they are immediately absorbed from the stomach into the bloodstream; and they are distributed to virtually every organ and tissue.

Grape seed extract also enhances capillary strength and vascular function, supporting the heart and decreasing bruising, edema (swelling) from injury or trauma, varicose veins and retinopathy.

By increasing peripheral circulation, OPCs may improve vision. Clinical studies have shown that antioxidants can halt cataract progression. OPCs, which have a strong affinity for the portion of the retina that is responsible for visual acuity, prevent free-radical damage and reinforce the collagen structures of the retina. Researchers have reported that OPCs improve symptoms of macular degeneration and other retinal diseases. Some health professionals believe that OPCs may also help in the prevention and treatment of glaucoma.

Finally, OPCs help reduce the aging of skin and loss of skin elasticity. Because of this, grape seed extract is often used topically in cosmetic preparations. Studies indicate that OPCs inhibit enzymes such as collagenase, elastase and hyaluronidase, all of which are involved in the breakdown of the skin's structural components. OPCs help protect the skin from ultraviolet radiation damage that leads to wrinkles and skin cancer; stabilize collagen and elastin; and help improve the elasticity and youthfulness of skin. They also strengthen the connective tissue of the skin and fat chambers. When that connection is broken, the quality of the skin changes (there is speculation that cellulite may actually be a sign of OPC deficiency). People taking grape seed extract have reported that it helps tone their skin and reduce cellulite, stretch marks and old scars.

## **Resveratrol**

Resveratrol is a fat-soluble polyphenol found in grapes and grape products (including grape seed extract). In 1992, scientists became aware of resveratrol in red wine, leading to speculation that resveratrol might be the answer to the French paradox. (The French paradox refers to the relatively low levels of heart disease among French people, despite their high consumption of saturated fat and cigarettes.) Since then, in vitro (test tube) studies have found resveratrol to have many potential health benefits.

## What Resveratrol Can Do for You

Scientists around the world have discovered many ways that resveratrol may benefit heart health. In 1995, Canadian researchers reported that resveratrol could protect against heart disease by reducing platelet aggregation, an early step in the development of blood clots that can lead to heart attacks or strokes. In 2002, German researchers found that resveratrol stimulates production of nitrous oxide, which helps relax arteries. In 2003, Italian researchers provided evidence that resveratrol could reduce the risk of atherosclerosis by keeping inflammatory cells from sticking to artery walls. Later that year, American researchers reported that resveratrol could slow the progression of atherosclerosis by inhibiting the spread of vascular smooth muscle cells.

Resveratrol may also play a role in cancer prevention, by inhibiting certain enzymes that activate some carcinogens and by promoting the excretion of other carcinogens. When cancer has already taken hold, resveratrol can arrest the cell cycle of cancer cells (allowing for DNA repair) and induce apoptosis (programmed cell death). Resveratrol can also inhibit cancer cell proliferation and angiogenesis, the process through which tumors support their growth by creating new blood vessels.

## Resveratrol and Bioavailability

In vitro studies have shown resveratrol to have many potent actions, and resveratrol is well absorbed in the gut; however, some researchers question whether the effects shown in the laboratory can take place in the body. In the May 2005 issue of the journal *Molecular Nutrition & Food Research*, scientists from the German Research Center of Food Chemistry wrote, "The oral bioavailability of resveratrol is almost zero due to rapid and extensive metabolism." In other words, very little resveratrol makes it into the blood.

The German researchers were not the first to discover this, however. In 2004, researchers at the Medical University of South Carolina acknowledged the low bioavailability of oral resveratrol, but suggested that resveratrol accumulates and provides benefits along the digestive tract. And in the November 2000 issue of the journal *Xenobiotica*, Italian researchers provided evidence that flavonoids and other components of grapes and wine improve the bioavailability of resveratrol.

Some researchers have taken a different approach to the problem of oral resveratrol bioavailability by skipping the stomach altogether. Using a delivery system known as PEGylated liposomes, supplements can deliver resveratrol through the mucous membranes in the mouth and directly to the blood. However, even resveratrol delivered directly to the blood is rapidly metabolized by the liver and removed from the blood in as little as 30 minutes.

However, low bioavailability does not mean resveratrol is useless; some researchers feel that it means investigators should shift their focus. For example, the previously mentioned German researchers suggest that future research focus on the effects of resveratrol metabolites.

## The Bottom Line

Grape seed extract contains powerful antioxidants and can reduce oxidation, strengthen and repair connective tissue and promote enzyme activity. It can also help moderate allergic and inflammatory responses by reducing histamine production. These actions help fight disease and boost your immune system. If you want to improve your chances against disease, enhance your health and fight the effects of aging, grape seed extract can help.

## GRAPE SEED EXTRACT AND RESVERATROL
## FAST FACTS

**Uses and Benefits:** Grape seed extract is an antioxidant, an anti-inflammatory, an antihistamine and an antiallergenic. It also improves circulation, promotes healing, restores collagen and strengthens weak blood vessels.

**Sources:** Grape seed extract is available at most health food stores. There are many different brands with different levels of active constituents, so ask your local supplement provider for recommendations.

Some of the beneficial nutrients in grape seed extract are also available in other foods. Resveratrol is found in grapes (and grape products such as red wine and purple grape juice), peanuts and some berries.

OPCs are found in many types of foods—usually in the peels, skins or seeds—but usually only in extremely small amounts. Some of the best sources are seasonal fruits such as grapes, blueberries, cherries and plums. Grape seeds contain the highest known concentration (95 percent) of OPCs, and pine bark the second highest (80 to 85 percent). Food processing and storage time reduce OPC bioavailability.

**Other Names:** Another name for the OPC complex is Pycnogenol. This was the name originally given to the complex by Dr. Jacques Masquelier, the first to scientifically discover OPCs. Dr. Masquelier patented the process of extracting OPCs from the bark of maritime pine trees, and Pycnogenol is now a trademarked name for OPC products extracted from pine bark.

# 8

# Green Tea

For thousands of years, green tea has been popular throughout Asia for its pleasant, soothing taste and time-honored health benefits. Practitioners of traditional Chinese medicine have recommended green tea since 3000 BC, and green tea is still an important part of the Chinese materia medica.

Modern studies confirm the efficacy of green tea for preventing and treating diseases and other health conditions. Green tea gets its health-promoting properties from phytochemicals known as polyphenols. Polyphenols are bitter, astringent phytochemicals that constitute 15 to 30 percent of dried green tea leaves by weight.

Although black tea is made from the same plant as green tea (*Camellia sinensis*), it does not provide the same health benefits. Black tea leaves are fermented, a process that that destroys polyphenols. Green tea leaves are lightly steamed, a process that protects polyphenols by destroying the enzyme that oxidizes them.

The polyphenols in fresh tea leaves are catechins, including gallocatechin (GC), epigallocatechin (EGC), epicatechin (EC), epigallocatechin gallate (EGCG) and epicatechin gallate (ECG). Catechins promote health in the following ways:

- Combating oxidative stress
- Protecting against cancer
- Lowering cholesterol levels
- Reducing blood pressure
- Fighting bacteria and viruses
- Protecting cognitive function

## Combating Oxidative Stress

Oxygen is essential for human life, but oxygen metabolism creates harmful by-products known as free radicals. Free radicals are unstable molecules that attack cells in the body, destroying cell membranes, damaging DNA and oxidizing lipids. These cellular assaults can contribute to cancer, heart disease and other serious health conditions. Our bodies protect themselves against free radicals with the help of antioxidants, which can be found in foods such as fresh fruits and vegetables—and green tea.

Studies demonstrate that the polyphenols in green tea efficiently scavenge free radicals and are more powerful than vitamins C and E, two well-known antioxidants. These polyphenols are particularly important in preventing lipid peroxidation, a process that plays a key role in the buildup of arterial plaque. Green tea also increases the activity of the body's own antioxidant system, including the activation of powerful natural antioxidants like superoxide dismutase and glutathione peroxidase.

# Protecting Against Cancer

The anticancer properties of green tea are largely the result of the ability of polyphenols to block the formation of carcinogenic compounds in the body. In addition, polyphenols trap and detoxify enzymes that produce carcinogens, rendering them harmless and inhibiting the spread of cancer cells. EGCG (the most common catechin in green tea) contributes to the programmed death of cancer cells before they can multiply and begin forming tumors.

Green tea appears to be most effective against cancers of the gastrointestinal tract, including stomach cancer, small intestine cancer, pancreatic cancer and colon cancer; lung cancer; and estrogen-related cancers, including breast cancer. The Japanese custom of drinking green tea with meals is thought to be a major factor in the low rates of these types of cancer in Japan.

# Lowering Cholesterol Levels

Cholesterol is essential for life, but it is also a major factor in the development of cardiovascular disease. There are basically two types of cholesterol: HDL ("good" cholesterol) and LDL ("bad" cholesterol). LDL cholesterol deposits cholesterol in the arteries; HDL cholesterol removes it. When too much LDL cholesterol circulates in the blood, it accumulates in the arteries, leading to atherosclerosis—hardening of the arteries. Atherosclerosis, especially in conjunction with high blood pressure, is a prime risk factor for heart disease. Compounds in green tea have been shown to reduce levels of bad LDL cholesterol and increase levels of good HDL cholesterol, thus helping to prevent atherosclerosis and heart disease.

In 1992, Japanese researchers examined the health records of 1,306 male retirees and discovered an inverse relationship between green tea consumption and serum cholesterol levels; in other words, men who drank more green tea had less cholesterol in their blood. Five years later, researchers in Hong Kong tested the effects of a variety of tea extracts on lipid profiles in rats. They reported that Chinese green tea decreased cholesterol levels without affecting HDL cholesterol levels, thus improving HDL ratios.

## Reducing Blood Pressure

High blood pressure (hypertension) is a serious risk factor for heart disease, stroke and other cardiovascular diseases. Some risk factors for hypertension—such as age, race and family history—can't be controlled. However, many major risk factors—such as poor diet, obesity and lack of exercise—are lifestyle related. Green tea consumption, it appears, is one lifestyle choice that can reduce the risk of hypertension.

In 1995, Japanese researchers published the results of a study on the effects of green tea on blood pressure in rats. The researchers gave rats green tea, water or a specially processed green tea with a high concentration of gamma-aminobutyric acid (GABA, a naturally occurring amino acid–like substance). In the *American Journal of Hypertension*, the researchers reported that the GABA-rich green tea lowered blood pressure in rats with preexisting hypertension and protected healthy rats against blood-pressure increases caused by a high-salt diet.

That these findings might apply in humans was supported by the results of a large study published in 2004 in the *Archives of Internal Medicine*. Researchers in Taiwan surveyed the tea-drinking habits of 1,507 patients with newly diagnosed hypertension. They found that habitual tea drinkers—those who drank at least 120 milliliters of tea daily for at least one year—were 46 percent less likely to develop hypertension than non-habitual tea drinkers. Those who drank more than 600 milliliters of tea daily were 65 percent less likely to develop hypertension.

## Fighting Bacteria and Viruses

In 2007, researchers in Slovenia reported that green tea catechins fight bacteria by attacking DNA gyrase, an enzyme necessary for bacterial reproduction and the target of many antibiotics. Other studies demonstrate more specific antibacterial applications for green tea. At a 2005 symposium of the American Chemical Society, researchers provided evidence that green tea extract kills several common food-borne bacteria, including salmonella. The results of a 2001 study in the *Journal of Medical Microbiology* show that green tea fights *Streptococcus mutans* and *Streptococcus sobrinus* bacteria, both of which contribute to tooth decay. And in 2003, researchers at Pace University in New York reported using green tea to inhibit the growth of bacteria responsible for strep throat and tooth decay.

Green tea also has antiviral properties. Researchers from South Korea's Yonsei University investigated the effects of green tea catechins on the influenza virus. According to the results of their study, published in 2005 in the journal *Antiviral Research*, two catechins, epigallocatechin gallate (EGCG) and epicatechin gallate (ECG), inhibited viral reproduction. In 2008, Chinese researchers published a study in the same journal showing that green tea extract inhibited the hepatitis B virus in laboratory settings.

# Protecting Against Cognitive Impairment

In a study published in the *American Journal of Clinical Nutrition* in 2006, researchers surveyed a group of 1,003 subjects over the age of 70 about their green tea consumption. After comparing the survey data against the rate of cognitive decline experienced by the study's participants, the authors wrote, "The prevalence of cognitive impairment decreased with increasing frequency of tea consumption." They concluded that "higher consumption of green tea is associated with lower prevalence of cognitive impairment in humans." While more research needs to be done in this area, initial results are promising.

# The Bottom Line

Because of the wide-ranging health benefits of green tea on so many different systems in the body, it makes sense to drink green tea and take green tea supplements to promote and preserve good health.

# GREEN TEA FAST FACTS

**Uses and Benefits:** Green tea acts as an antioxidant, helps protect against cancer, fights bacterial infections and tooth decay, lowers cholesterol levels and may delay the onset of atherosclerosis.

**Sources:** The most common source of green tea is an infusion made from tea bags or loose tea leaves. Green tea extracts and capsules are also widely available.

**Special Considerations:** Drink green tea without milk, which may bind with some beneficial compounds in the tea and make them unavailable to the body. Some experts suggest drinking four to 10 cups of green tea a day; if this seems like too much, consider a green tea supplement. Be aware that green tea contains small quantities of caffeine.

Black tea does not offer the same health benefits as green tea. Unlike green tea leaves, which are gently steamed, black tea is fermented, a process that destroys polyphenols.

# 9

# Multivitamin/Mineral Supplements

If you were to take only one of the many dietary supplements available today, which would it be? Many nutrition experts recommend a high-quality multivitamin/mineral supplement (referred to simply as a multivitamin, or multi). A good multivitamin will provide you with a wide variety of nutrients that are necessary for the basic functioning of your body, and current scientific research reveals that many of the nutrients in multivitamins can also help prevent disease and promote well-being.

How important is a daily multivitamin? Consider this: In 2002, the American Medical Association published a recommendation that all adults take a daily multivitamin, because many Americans, especially women and high-risk groups (such as the elderly and those with chronic health conditions), don't receive adequate levels of essential nutrients from their diets.

You may be thinking that there's nothing revolutionary about multivitamins; after all, they've been around for years. In a time when thousands of products line the supermarket shelves, daily news stories bombard us with miraculous health claims and slick infomercials tempt us with promises of instant results, a simple multivitamin may seem a little . . . well, simple. But for those who want to prevent nutritional deficiencies and boost overall health, there's no better way to start than with a high-quality multivitamin.

No supplement—not even the best multivitamin—can replace a healthful diet of whole grains, legumes, fresh fruits and vegetables, lean meats, fish and healthy fats. However, many experts agree that the standard American diet (SAD) does not typically provide all of the nutrients our bodies need. Many factors—including over-processed foods, busy schedules, and modern agricultural practices, which reduce the nutrient content of some foods—make it difficult for most of us to get adequate amounts of all the nutrients our bodies need to function at optimal levels.

A high-quality multivitamin may be the best health insurance your money can buy, for several reasons:

- A multivitamin can guarantee that a less-than-perfect diet will not put you at risk for nutrient deficiencies and the health problems those deficiencies may create.
- Most multivitamins provide high levels of certain nutrients that are known to offer additional benefits at levels above what diet alone can provide; levels that also exceed the U.S. government's reference daily intakes (RDIs), which many nutritional experts consider to be marginally adequate, at best.
- Multivitamins are convenient. Many people find it confusing, cumbersome and inconvenient to take a handful of pills each day to cover their nutritional needs; taking a single multivitamin tablet takes but a few seconds.

Multivitamins are even good for future generations: researchers at the University of North Carolina at Chapel Hill have found that that women who take multivitamins prior to becoming pregnant have a lower risk of preterm births.

# Choosing a Multi

When you go to choose a multivitamin, the selection can be overwhelming. You'll find dozens of different brands, several different forms (tablets, capsules, powders, liquids, chewables, etc.), widely varying ingredients, and a huge range of prices. But don't despair. The following section provides the basic information you'll need to select a high-quality multivitamin that suits your needs and fits your budget.

## Where to Purchase

Multivitamins are available in health food stores, grocery stores, drug stores and warehouse stores, as well as from Web sites and mail-order retailers. When first selecting a multivitamin, visit a reputable health food store in your area. Most health food stores offer a wide range of products to meet individual needs, are staffed by well-trained and knowledgeable employees, and have good product turnover to ensure that the supplements they sell are fresh. Also, health food stores value their customers and will be willing to work with you if you purchase products that for some reason don't meet your needs.

If you purchase supplements from drug stores or pharmacies, you will typically find a more limited selection, but many pharmacists are knowledgeable enough about supplements to help steer you in the right direction.

## How Much to Spend

Consider various factors when deciding how much to spend on a multivitamin. Do a little research and compare the prices of the products you're considering. If most supplements cost more than 10 dollars and you find one that sells for only three dollars, you may want to pass on the cheaper one. But remember, more expensive doesn't always mean better, and cheaper doesn't always mean less effective.

For those whose primary concern is price, warehouse clubs like Costco and Sam's Club offer multivitamins at substantial discounts, as do various Web sites. You may want to visit a health food store and talk to the staff to determine the right multivitamin for you, and then buy a starter package of the product. If you can't afford to continue buying that particular supplement from the health food store, you may be able to find the same product online at a substantial discount.

## Determining Quality

Look for multivitamins from manufacturers that conduct quality control tests. It's comforting to know that a manufacturer verifies and tests raw materials. Also look for products that that have been tested for purity and potency. This means that if a label says that a product contains 500 milligrams of vitamin C, the company has actually tested that product batch instead of relying on other calculations. Most manufacturers provide their Web address or phone number on their labels, and you may want to contact the company to learn more about the specific quality control tests they perform.

## USP Approved

Look for products that bear the USP logo. USP is the abbreviation for *United States Pharmacopeia*, an official public standards–setting authority for health care products in the United States. Their seal tells you that the multivitamin has been tested and approved for adequate nutrient absorption. While many excellent products aren't tested by the USP, the USP logo is one indicator that your product will dissolve and be absorbed properly.

## Labels and Packaging

Examine the packaging of the multivitamin you're considering. Choose a product with legible labels: the front panel should provide the name and quantity of the product, and the side panels should provide nutritional information and an ingredient list with the exact quantity of each ingredient. Also, look for products that provide the manufacturer's contact information, a lot number, an expiration date and clear instructions.

## Recommendations from Store Staff

If you're not sure about which product to choose, don't be afraid to ask! Staff members at reputable health food stores are well trained and knowledgeable about the products they sell. Pay attention to their recommendations, which are often based on positive feedback from other customers.

# What Should My Multivitamin Contain?

There are no perfect answers about what an ideal multivitamin should contain. Whether you're a man, woman or child will help determine the product that's best for you, as will your age, your dietary habits and the like. You may also need to take some nutrients as separate supplements, since multivitamins don't always provide adequate quantities of some nutrients (for example, most multivitamins contain minimal quantities of calcium, because the full RDI of calcium is simply too bulky to fit into a single multivitamin pill). The following are some suggestions for nutrients to look for in a good multivitamin:

## Vitamin A and Beta-carotene

Look for a product with more beta-carotene than vitamin A. Beta-carotene is a precursor to vitamin A (meaning the body converts it into vitamin A as needed). It's far less toxic in large quantities, and it can be utilized by the body as needed. Moreover, it appears that beta-carotene offers more protection against cancer than vitamin A.

### Benefits of Vitamin A
- Assists in bone development and growth
- Acts as a cofactor in essential enzyme reactions
- Supports healthy testicular and ovarian function
- Enables normal retinal function

## Vitamin C

Vitamin C is an important antioxidant that should be supplied at levels well above the minimum requirements (60 milligrams). Some prominent researchers, such as two-time Nobel Prize winner Linus Pauling (1901–1994), advocate taking huge amounts of vitamin C—tens of thousands of milligrams daily—while others suggest a more moderate 700 to 1,500 milligrams a day. Higher daily intake may only temporarily raise blood levels of vitamin C, though this could be beneficial. If you want to take more vitamin C than your multivitamin provides, you can easily take a separate supplement.

## *Benefits of Vitamin C*

- Prevents and treats scurvy
- Acts as a powerful antioxidant
- Assists in iron absorption
- Helps treat anemia
- Promotes collagen growth in connective tissue
- Helps wounds and broken bones heal
- Treats urinary tract infections

## *Bioflavonoids*

Many multivitamin formulas contain bioflavonoids, which are thought to enhance the action of vitamin C. Research shows that bioflavonoids also help reduce the risk of certain diseases.

## *Benefits of Bioflavonoids*

- Help metabolize carbohydrates and amino acids
- Assist in formation of fatty acids
- Support healthy blood cells, hair, skin, nerves, bones and male reproductive organs

## *Vitamin E*

Vitamin E is an important antioxidant that should be supplied at levels well above the RDI of 30 IU (international units) per day. Many authorities recommend 200 to 1,000 IU per day to help prevent age-related degenerative diseases such as cancer and atherosclerosis. Experts recommend that elderly people with risk factors for heart disease and those suffering from Alzheimer's-related dementia take extra vitamin E. Most natural health care providers prefer the natural d-alpha form of vitamin E over the chemically synthesized dl-alpha form.

## Benefits of Vitamin E

- Acts as a powerful antioxidant
- Prevents deficiency in low-weight infants
- Acts as an anti-clotting agent
- Assists in the formation of red blood cells

## Vitamin K

Vitamin K is included in multivitamin formulas because it can help prevent bone loss. A daily dose of 80 to 300 micrograms conforms to current RDI standards. Vitamin K is especially important for patients with a history of intestinal malabsorption or chronic antibiotic therapy (antibiotics kill vitamin K–producing intestinal bacteria).

## Benefits of Vitamin K

- Helps prevent abnormal bleeding
- Promotes normal growth and development
- Helps prevent bone loss

## B-Complex Vitamins

The B vitamin family includes eight distinct vitamins:

- B1—Thiamine
- B2—Riboflavin
- B3—Niacin
- B5—Pantothenic Acid

- B6—Pyridoxine
- B7—Biotin
- B9—Folic Acid
- B12—Cyanocobalamin

Each B vitamin is a separately functioning coenzyme that affects a wide-range of processes and functions in the human body. If you have a specific condition for which a single B vitamin is known to be helpful, a separate supplement of this vitamin may be added to a multi, preferably after consultation with a knowledgeable health care provider. See the chapter on B-complex vitamins for specific benefits of each B vitamin.

## Vitamin D

We get vitamin D from two sources: our food and the sun. Vitamin D deficiency has been linked to higher risks of colorectal and breast cancer, so it's important to guarantee an adequate intake. In fact, vitamin D was recently shown to reduce the risk of polyp development in the colon, a precursor to colon cancer. For those who don't get regular exposure to sunlight or eat vitamin D–fortified foods, 400 IU per day may be optimal. Because vitamin D plays a role in bone building, people with an increased risk for osteoporosis may benefit from 800 IU per day.

### Benefits of Vitamin D

- Prevents rickets
- Treats low blood calcium in cases of kidney disease
- Helps promote bone formation
- Promotes normal development of children and infants

## Calcium

Since calcium is such a bulky mineral, manufacturers include only a portion of the RDI in a typical multivitamin. Because calcium plays an important role in bone building, muscle contraction and more, it's important to ensure adequate intake from your diet. Some people, especially women, who have a greater risk of osteoporosis, may need an additional calcium supplement. When choosing calcium, as part of a multivitamin or as an individual supplement, look for the calcium-citrate form.

### Benefits of Calcium

- Promotes normal growth and development
- Helps prevent osteoporosis
- Builds strong bones and teeth
- Maintains strength and density of bones
- Helps the body utilize amino acids
- Helps prevent muscle cramps

## Magnesium

Magnesium is essential for the use of calcium, and the two work hand-in-hand in the body. Some experts believe that magnesium deficiencies are more common than previously thought because so many factors interfere with magnesium absorption, including prolonged stress, consumption of coffee and soft drinks, taking diuretics and eating too much fat. Magnesium deficiencies can cause insulin resistance and can negatively affect smooth muscles and platelets, increasing the risk of hypertension. Magnesium deficiency has also been linked to dozens of other conditions, such as migraines, premenstrual syndrome, recurrent bacterial and fungal infections, muscle cramps and Alzheimer's disease.

## *Benefits of Magnesium*

- Assists in bone formation
- Supports normal function of nervous system
- Regulates normal heart rhythm
- Strengthens tooth enamel
- Helps maintain stable metabolism

## *Potassium*

Multivitamins often include potassium at doses around 100 milligrams per tablet, far below the recommended intake of 3,000 milligrams or more. However, individuals with varied, healthful diets usually don't have a problem obtaining adequate amounts of potassium.

## *Benefits of Potassium*

- Promotes regular heartbeat
- Maintains water balance in body tissues
- Supports normal muscle contraction
- Treats drug-induced potassium deficiency
- Promotes transfer of nutrients to cells

## **Zinc and Copper**

Zinc and copper work together in the human body, so a good multivitamin should contain adequate quantities of both. A 15:1 zinc-to-copper ratio is considered ideal, with a range of 10 to 30 parts zinc to one part copper being acceptable.

### Benefits of Copper

- Promotes formation of red blood cells
- Helps produce enzymes needed for respiration
- Assists in the formation of hemoglobin in red blood cells

### Benefits of Zinc

- Strong antioxidant properties
- Helps wounds heal
- Assists in the synthesis of RNA and DNA
- Promotes the division, repair, and growth of cells

## Manganese

Manganese has received a lot of attention for its role in bone and joint health. Most multivitamins provide only a few milligrams of manganese—enough to satisfy the minimum requirements—but you may want to look for one that provides more than the minimum or consider taking a separate trace mineral supplement.

### Benefits of Manganese

- Promotes normal growth and development
- Assists enzymes in generating energy
- Promotes normal cellular function

## Chromium

Chromium is important in sugar and lipid metabolism and should be included in any complete multivitamin formula. However, some manufacturers include far less than the recommended 50 to 200 micrograms in their product's daily dose. Organically bound chromium is much better absorbed than inorganic chromium chloride.

## Benefits of Chromium

- Assists insulin in the regulation of blood sugar
- Improves glucose tolerance in people with type 2 diabetes
- Promotes healthy glucose metabolism

## Selenium

Selenium is an important antioxidant cofactor and may be important in cancer prevention. A new RDI has been established at 70 micrograms, but many formulas contain as much as 200 micrograms, which some authorities consider to be in the upper range of recommended intakes.

## Benefits of Selenium

- Acts as a powerful antioxidant
- Teams up with vitamin E for additional antioxidant properties
- Promotes normal growth and development

## Other Nutrients

Multivitamins vary widely in their nutritional composition. Many include trace minerals such as boron, molybdenum and vanadium. While there are no established recommendations for these nutrients, experts agree that they're necessary for good health. If your multivitamin doesn't contain trace minerals, consider taking an occasional trace mineral supplement.

# The Bottom Line

As we said at the beginning, if you were to take only one dietary supplement, a good multivitamin would be your best bet. Many of us aren't getting optimal levels of all the essential nutrients, but a multivitamin can ensure that our nutritional needs are met. The multivitamin/mineral supplement could now replace the apple in a new adage, "A multi a day keeps the doctor away."

---

## MULTIVITAMIN/MINERAL FAST FACTS

**Product forms:** Tablets, capsules, liquid, powder and chewables.

Uses and Benefits: Multivitamin supplements prevent nutrient deficiencies and help maintain basic body functions and processes. Multivitamin supplements may also help prevent health conditions such as heart disease, diabetes, cancer and arthritis.

**Special Considerations:** Always consult with a qualified health care provider before taking a dietary supplement to help treat a specific disease or condition.

# 10

# Nattokinase

Perhaps you've heard about nattokinase, a natural enzyme that recent studies have shown to have anticoagulant properties. Perhaps you'd like to know more.

Any discussion of nattokinase must begin with a discussion of natto. To the uninitiated, natto—a sticky, smelly dish of fermented soybeans—is intimidating. But in Japan, natto has been a staple in traditional diets for thousands of years.

Traditionally, natto was made by soaking soybeans in water and then steaming them before finally mixing the beans with rice straw and allowing the mixture to ferment for 24 hours. When *Bacillus natto*, a bacterium found in rice straw, combines with the soybeans, nattokinase is born. Without the bacteria, natto would be just another bowl of stinky beans.

In the early twentieth century, researchers discovered a way to introduce *B. natto* to the soybeans without using straw, therefore simplifying the process of making natto and producing more consistent results.

With its sticky appearance and strong odor (if you like blue cheese, you'll love natto), natto is an acquired taste, and even in Japan natto consumption is mostly limited to the eastern region of Kanto. But despite its smell and appearance, natto has a surprisingly mild taste and has been used in Japan for ages as a folk remedy to treat heart and vascular diseases as well as fatigue and beriberi. Even Japanese pets, who don't seem to mind the smell and texture, have enjoyed natto as an ingredient in their food, and it has allegedly improved their health. However, the scope and degree of the benefits of nattokinase were not documented until fairly recently.

## Nattokinase and Blood Clots

While studying physiological chemistry at the University of Chicago Medical School, Japanese researcher Dr. Hiroyuki Sumi wanted to find a natural enzyme that would help dissolve blood clots, which are associated with heart attacks and strokes. Because heart disease and stroke are the first and third most common causes of death in the United States and account for more deaths than all cancers and injuries combined, discovering a natural supplement that prevents cardiovascular disease would be a great leap forward. Even more so if that supplement had already been in use for thousands of years and provided a number of additional benefits.

In 1980, Dr. Sumi tested over 173 natural foods as part of his research. You can imagine his joy when he dropped natto in a Petri dish containing fibrin (a protein involved in the clotting of blood) and the natto completely dissolved the fibrin within 18 hours.

Fibrin is a natural protein in our blood that helps blood clot in response to injury or trauma. The clotting process is vital; however, problems occur when the body is unable to completely break down the clots after they have served their purpose.

The body produces more than 20 enzymes to create blood clots, but only one—plasmin—to eliminate them. If the body produces too little plasmin, it cannot completely dissolve blood clots, and fragments will flow through the bloodstream, damaging blood vessel linings and sometimes blocking blood vessels completely.

Blood carries oxygen throughout the body. If a blood clot cuts off that oxygen supply, tissues will eventually die. A blood clot in the heart can cause angina and heart attacks. A blood clot in the brain can cause a stroke.

Nattokinase, which dissolves fibrin and stimulates the body's production of plasmin, seems to clean up old blood clots that would otherwise circulate through the bloodstream and damage blood vessels. This is in contrast to current pharmaceutical drugs, which inhibit platelet aggregation, interfering with the blood's normal ability to clot.

"In some ways, nattokinase is actually superior to conventional clot-dissolving drugs," said Dr. Milner of the Center for Natural Medicine in Portland, Oregon. "T-PAs [tissue plasminogen activators] like urokinase [an anti-clotting agent] are only effective when taken intravenously and often fail simply because a stroke or heart-attack victim's arteries have been hardened beyond the point where they can be treated by any other clot-dissolving agent. Nattokinase, however, can help prevent that hardening."

Aging patients are the most likely to benefit from the blood-thinning effects of nattokinase. As the body ages, plasmin production decreases, making the blood more likely to clot and increasing the risk of heart attack or stroke. Nattokinase will be most beneficial

## RISK FACTORS FOR CARDIOVASCULAR DISEASE

Risk factors are traits that indicate a person's likelihood to develop a disease. The more risk factors you have, the greater your risk. While some factors are hereditary, you can control many others. The following are common risk factors for cardiovascular disease:

- High cholesterol
- Family history
- High blood pressure
- Excess body weight
- Smoking
- Physical inactivity

to those who suffer from conditions involving clogged arteries; for example, patients with senile dementia caused by blocked cerebral arteries.

In a recent human study, researchers from JCR Pharmaceuticals, Oklahoma State University and Miyazaki Medical College (in Japan) tested nattokinase on 12 healthy Japanese volunteers—six women and six men between the ages of 21 and 55. The researchers gave the volunteers seven ounces of natto before breakfast and then tracked the volunteers' fibrinolytic activity (or breakdown of fibrin) through a series of blood tests.

In one test, the researchers took a blood sample and artificially induced a clot. Within two hours of treatment, the time needed to dissolve clots in the blood of patients who had received nattokinase was half of what it was in the blood of patients who had not received nattokinase. The increased ability to dissolve blood clots lasted for up to eight hours.

In another study, Dr. Sumi's team conducted a test on two groups of dogs: one group received nattokinase tablets and the other group received a placebo. The researchers then created a clot in each dog, completely blocking a major leg vein. Within five hours, circulation had been completely restored in the nattokinase-fed dogs; in contrast,

---

**TIPS TO REDUCE YOUR RISK OF CARDIOVASCULAR DISEASE**

- Stop smoking
- Exercise
- Eat a diet rich in whole-grain foods and fiber
- Drink eight to 10 glasses of water per day
- Engage in regular strength training
- Practice stress-reduction techniques

---

the placebo-fed dogs still had a complete vein blockage 18 hours later.

In 1995, Japanese researchers tested nattokinase's ability to dissolve blood clots in the carotid arteries of rats. Animals treated with nattokinase regained 62 percent of blood flow, while those treated with plasmin regained only 15.8 percent of blood flow.

In 2003, researchers from the Hamamatsu University School of Medicine induced endothelial (the inner lining of blood vessels) damage in the femoral arteries of rats that had been given nattokinase. Under normal circumstances, blood clotting and a thickening of arterial walls would occur; however, the fibrinolytic activity of nattokinase suppressed both.

## Nattokinase and Blood Pressure

Natto has been used as a traditional folk medicine in Japan to treat high blood pressure, and recent studies confirm this benefit. In 1995, researchers at Japan's Miyazaki Medical College and Kurashiki University of Science and Arts studied the effects of nattokinase on high blood pressure in both animals and humans.

In one study, researchers gave volunteers with high blood pressure

30 grams of natto extract (equivalent to seven ounces of natto) every day for four days. In four out of five volunteers, systolic blood pressure dropped an average of 10.9 percent and diastolic blood pressure dropped an average of 9.7 percent.

In another study, researchers gave natto extract to rats. According to the data, the rats experienced an average 12.7 percent drop in systolic blood pressure after just two hours.

## Retinal Vein Occlusion

In a 1994 case study, a team of researchers used nattokinase to treat a retinal vein occlusion. The blood vessels draining out of the eye of a 58-year-old Japanese man were blocked by a blood clot, and the blockage had caused bleeding and swelling in the eye, resulting in tiny vessels bursting. The researchers fed the man a 100-gram serving of natto—a rich source of nattokinase—before he went to bed every night. Ten days later, bleeding from the bottom of the man's eye had stopped. After 20 days, the man's vision recovered and he was sent home from the hospital with instructions to continue to eat natto twice a week. After two months, the occlusion had completely dissolved.

## Cholesterol

The body's natural response to an arterial-wall injury caused by blood clots is to build up cholesterol in arterial plaques. Hence, by preventing blood clots, nattokinase may help prevent elevated cholesterol levels.

# Diabetes

Certain types of diabetes have also been shown to be caused by changes in the blood vessels that supply the pancreas. These changes may be linked to small blood clots.

# Forms and Dosage

As mentioned earlier, natto is the original source of nattokinase. However, thanks to modern technology, nattokinase is available in capsule form. A variety of nattokinase supplements are currently available, including a highly advanced supplement that contains no soy and no vitamin K (which promotes blood clotting).

Doses of nattokinase are measured in fibrin units (FU). Standard dosage recommendations are 2,000 FU (50 grams) daily for preventive use and 4,000 to 6,000 FU (160 to 200 grams) daily for therapeutic use.

For safety, those who use nattokinase for therapeutic purposes should choose a high-quality, well-researched nattokinase enzyme that is standardized for potency and guaranteed to be free of vitamin K.

# Drug Interactions and Side Effects

Natto is a traditional food and is considered safe when eaten in moderate amounts. However, nattokinase enzymes and natto extracts that naturally contain vitamin K can interfere with blood-thinning drugs like warfarin and aspirin. People who are currently using blood thinners and those who suffer from kidney or liver disease should consult their doctor before using nattokinase.

People with bleeding disorders should not take nattokinase. People with ongoing bleeding problems, including ulcers, recent surgery or recent major trauma, should also avoid nattokinase.

Pregnant or nursing women should consult their doctors before using nattokinase until additional research confirms its safety.

# The Bottom Line

Though its natural source is stinky and slimy, nattokinase has demonstrated some remarkable health-promoting qualities. Chief among them is nattokinase's ability to improve circulatory health through its blood-thinning and anti-clotting properties. With heart disease and stroke among the most common killers in the United States, nattokinase may belong in your arsenal of disease-preventing supplements.

Could nattokinase be the next true breakthrough in cardiovascular health? Dr. Miler thinks so: "In all my years of research as a professor of cardiovascular and pulmonary medicine, natto and nattokinase represent the most exciting new development in the prevention and treatment of cardiovascular-related diseases," he said. "We have finally found a potent natural agent that can thin and dissolve clots effectively, and with relative safety and without side effects."

# NATTOKINASE FAST FACTS

**Uses and Benefits:** Nattokinase helps promote cardiovascular health by preventing blood clots and supporting healthy blood pressure and cholesterol levels. Nattokinase may also provide benefits for diabetics.

Sources: Natto is the only dietary source of nattokinase. Because natto is an acquired taste, most people will prefer nattokinase capsules. Look for supplements without vitamin K. Soy-free nattokinase supplements are available for those with food sensitivities.

**Special Considerations:** Vitamin K can interfere with the action of blood thinners like aspirin and warfarin, so people using these medications should avoid natto and nattokinase supplements with vitamin K. Do not use nattokinase if you have a bleeding disorder or if you have recently undergone surgery or experienced physical trauma. If you are pregnant, consult with your physician before using nattokinase.

# 11

# Natural Sweeteners

These days, sugar is public enemy number one, blamed for the epidemics of obesity, type 2 diabetes and more. But does sugar deserve its unfavorable reputation? And even if it does, who wants to go through life without indulging their sweet tooth?

Sugars—caloric sweeteners—can be divided into two groups: intrinsic sugars, such as lactose in dairy products and fructose in whole fruits; and added sugars, such as sucrose (table sugar), high fructose corn syrup and concentrated sugar sources such as honey, syrups and fruit concentrates.

Nutritionist Marion Nestle reports that from 1980 to 2004 the yearly supply of sugars in the United States increased from 120 pounds per person to 142 pounds per person. The U.S. Department of Agriculture (USDA) estimates the average American eats 31 teaspoons (five ounces) of sugar per day—that's more than two pounds per week! Sugar accounts for 500 calories per day in the average American diet, or 25 percent of average daily energy requirements.

Conventional wisdom tells us that so much sugar can't be good. Sugar is popularly associated with many of America's health problems,

## THE GLYCEMIC INDEX

Sharp increases in blood glucose (sugar) have been associated with type 2 diabetes, obesity, heart disease and cancer. To measure the impact of foods on blood sugar, scientists developed the glycemic index. The glycemic index is a measure of the increase in blood sugar after eating a particular food—the greater the increase, the higher the glycemic index. Only carbohydrates affect blood sugar levels, and fat and protein can lower the glycemic response. Pure glucose has a glycemic index of 100; in contrast, peanuts have a glycemic index of only 14.

Blood glucose levels are also affected by how much food is eaten. The combined effect of serving size and glycemic index on blood sugar is referred to as the glycemic load. Doubling the serving size of carbohydrates will double the glycemic load. To decrease your glycemic load and increase your health, eat mostly foods with a low glycemic index (such as whole grains, fruits, legumes and non-starchy vegetables) and avoid starchy foods (such as white rice, potatoes and white bread) and sugary foods (such as cookies, candy and soft drinks).

from hyperactivity to heart disease. But does science support these claims?

That depends on who you ask. In 2001, Anne Mardis of the Center for Nutrition Policy and Promotion (a division of the USDA) wrote a review of the available research on sugar intake and health. Conceding only that sugar was a cause—but not the only cause—of tooth decay, Mardis concluded, "Recent evidence shows that… the intake of added sugars is not directly related to diabetes, heart disease, obesity, and hyperactivity, as was previously thought."

Nestle disagrees, and she's not alone. In 2004, Jim Mann refuted Mardis' conclusions in *The Lancet*, the respected British medical journal. According to Mann, sugar may not directly cause chronic disease, but substantial evidence links sugar consumption to obesity, which contributes to coronary heart disease, type 2 diabetes and other chronic diseases. Also in 2004, a team of medical researchers linked type 2 diabetes to corn syrup and other refined carbohydrates.

Regardless of what it *does* do, sugar is notable for what it *doesn't* do; namely, provide the body with essential nutrients. Sugar calories are empty calories—they provide energy and nothing else. According to Nestle, "It is all too easy to eat sweeteners in prodigious amounts, driving healthier foods out of your diet, adding unneeded calories and forcing your metabolism to go into glycemic overload." Replacing sugar calories with healthier alternatives is a step towards better nutrition.

## Food Science to the Rescue?

The food industry has responded to the demand for sugar alternatives with a variety of calorie-free artificial sweeteners. Some of the most popular include aspartame (NutraSweet, Equal), saccharin (Sweet'N Low, SugarTwin), acesulfame potassium (Sunett, Sweet One) and sucralose (Splenda). These sweeteners are common ingredients in diet soft drinks, low-fat yogurt products, sugar-free candy and more. Theoretically, artificial sweeteners, which are calorie free and have no glycemic impact, avoid many of the pitfalls associated with sugar.

However, many consumers are wary of artificial ingredients, and artificial sweeteners are no exception. A study from the 1970s reported a connection between saccharin and bladder cancer in rats. Although the mechanism responsible for this connection does not occur in people, concern about artificial sweeteners lives on. A quick Internet search reveals numerous Web sites claiming connections between artificial sweeteners and cancer, toxicity and more.

Clinical evidence suggests that there is no link between artificial sweeteners and cancer. (In 2006, scientists at the National Cancer Institute determined that aspartame did not cause cancer in humans, despite an earlier study reporting a link between aspartame and cancer in rats). This is not, however, to say that artificial sweeteners are free of consequences. In 2007, a team of researchers published a study in the journal *Circulation* that linked increased soft drink consumption with metabolic syndrome (a collection of risk factors such as obesity, high blood pressure and impaired glucose tolerance). Surprisingly, this connection also applied to those who drank artificially sweetened diet soft drinks. Clearly, the health consequences of artificial sweeteners are not yet fully understood.

# Natural Alternatives

Fortunately, there are alternatives for those who wish to reduce their sugar consumption without sacrificing sweetness or resorting to artificial additives. Health food stores sell many caloric and non-caloric natural sweeteners. While not technically supplements, these sweeteners have a place in every health-conscious kitchen.

## Stevia

Stevia is a perennial shrub native to regions of South America. In traditional Brazilian and Paraguayan medical systems, the stevia leaf was used to treat diabetes, obesity, tooth decay, high blood pressure, fatigue, depression and more. But modern interest in stevia has little to do with the plant's medicinal properties.

Interest in stevia centers on stevioside, a chemical constituent that is 300 times sweeter than table sugar and essentially calorie free.

Indigenous tribes in Brazil and Paraguay have used stevia as a sweetener for centuries. During World War II, the British used stevia when their supply of sugar was cut off. And Japanese food processors have used stevia to prepare pickled foods since the early 1970s. However, in 1991 the FDA banned stevia as a food additive, and regulatory agencies in Canada and the European Union have done likewise.

Regulators argue that stevia may cause reproductive problems and cancer and interfere with energy metabolism. But stevia supporters disagree. According to herbalist Daniel Mowrey, "Few substances have ever yielded such consistently negative results in toxicity trials as have stevia. Almost every toxicity test imaginable has been performed on stevia extract or stevioside at one time or another. The results are always negative." Furthermore, there have been no reports of adverse effects in Japan and other countries where stevia is used as a sweetener.

Stevia may not be available as a food additive, but it is available as a dietary supplement. Stevia supplements are sold as whole leaves, capsules, liquids and powders. Liquids and powders are the best for use as sweeteners. Remember, stevia is extremely sweet, so only a small amount is necessary (three to four teaspoons of stevia powder provide the sweetness of one cup of sugar).

The FDA may lift its ban on stevia soon; in December 2008, the FDA approved stevia-derived sweeteners developed by PepsiCo and the Coca-Cola Company, and further approval may follow. But even if the ban remains in place, you can still enjoy stevia in your own home. Just remember—a little stevia goes a long way.

## Xylitol

Xylitol belongs to a class of caloric sweeteners known as sugar alcohols. Sugar alcohols are naturally occurring carbohydrates derived from the fibers of fruits, vegetables and other plants. Because they are not completely metabolized in the body, sugar alcohols provide fewer calories than sugar. And because they require little—if any—insulin to metabolize them, sugar alcohols have a low glycemic impact.

Emil Fischer, a German chemist, discovered xylitol in 1891. Xylitol has been used as a sweetener since the 1960s. It is as sweet as sucrose and has no unpleasant aftertaste. Unlike sucrose, which provides four calories per gram, xylitol provides only 2.4 calories per gram.

Xylitol is a common ingredient in chewing gum and toothpaste, as well as in mints, candies, mouthwashes, cough syrups, multivitamins and more. Several brands offer xylitol powder for cooking and baking.

Studies first suggested that xylitol might benefit oral health in 1970. Since then, research has shown that xylitol fights cavity-causing bacteria, reduces plaque and prevents tooth demineralization. In 1995, researchers from the University of Michigan published the results of a 40-month double-blind study showing that xylitol chewing gum can reduce rates of dental cavities. In 2006, citing this study and others, the American Academy of Pediatric Dentistry (AAPD) recommended xylitol for long-term cavity prevention. According to the AAPD, the ideal dose of xylitol is four to ten grams per day, divided into three to seven servings.

The American Diabetes Association approves of xylitol as a sweetener for people with diabetes. However, xylitol is low-glycemic, not non-glycemic; therefore, diabetics must still control their xylitol consumption, as should everyone else—because xylitol is not broken down completely in the intestines, large quantities may cause diarrhea.

## Agave Syrup

As a source of food, the cactus-like agave is nothing new. For thousands of years, native Mexicans consumed agave nectar, which they referred to as the "nectar of the gods." Later, the Spaniards used the plant to produce tequila. Today, agave syrup is gaining popularity as an alternative sweetener.

Agave syrup, which has a slightly runnier consistency than honey, is nearly three times as sweet as sucrose. Even so, agave syrup scores low on the glycemic index, releasing energy into the bloodstream slowly rather than causing a quick spike (and subsequent crash). The glycemic index of agave syrup is between 11 and 19—much lower than sucrose (58 to 110) and honey (32 to 58). This is because agave syrup is composed primarily of fructose, the same natural sugar that gives fresh fruit its sweetness.

Agave syrup also contains inulin, a prebiotic that may support healthy bacteria in the intestines.

Most health food stores sell both light and dark agave syrup. Light agave syrup has been filtered and has a neutral flavor. Dark, unfiltered agave syrup has more minerals and a distinctive vanilla-like flavor.

Agave is delicious on fruits and cereals and dissolved into hot drinks. Agave can even be used for baking—just replace one cup of sugar with one third of a cup of agave syrup.

## Luo Han Guo

For thousands of years, luo han guo has been used as a food and a traditional healing herb. Luo han guo is a small fruit native to southern China, where both the dried fruit and the powdered extract play an important role in daily life.

Traditionally, luo han guo was used to purify the blood and treat cold symptoms and gastrointestinal disorders. Today, preliminary research suggests that luo han guo may protect against cancer. In 2002, an article in the journal *Pure and Applied Chemistry* reported that mogroside V, a component of luo han guo, inhibited skin cancer in mice. In 2003, researchers from Japan's Kyoto University attributed the same effect to different constituents of luo han guo called glycosides.

Despite the potential health benefits of luo han guo, most interest lies in the culinary use of the fruit. Luo han guo extract is reported to be 150 to 300 times as sweet as sugar. Because it dissolves in water and retains its flavor when cooked, luo han guo is a suitable alternative to artificial sweeteners.

Luo han guo extract is calorie free and does not raise blood sugar levels. In addition, luo han guo may prevent maltose (a carbohydrate found in grains such as barley) from raising blood sugar levels. In 2005, Japanese researchers published a study on the effects of luo han guo extract on blood glucose levels in rats. The researchers observed that the extract inhibited blood sugar increases when given to rats three minutes before an oral dose of maltose. However, the researchers observed no such effect when the rats were given glucose. These findings suggest that luo han guo extract may inhibit maltase, the enzyme responsible for metabolizing maltose.

## Bottom Line

Sugar is delicious, but its consequences aren't so sweet. Fortunately, there are alternatives. Look to nature instead of the laboratory next time you crave something sweet, and support your health along with your sweet tooth.

## NATURAL SWEETENERS FAST FACTS

**Uses and Benefits:** Natural sweeteners can satisfy any sweet tooth without causing a blood-sugar spike or relying on potentially dangerous chemicals. Additionally, xylitol may support oral health, and luo han guo may offer some protection against cancer.

**Sources:** Stevia is available in whole-leaf form or in capsules, liquids and powders. Xylitol is a common ingredient in chewing gum, toothpaste, candy and more. Some brands offer xylitol powder for kitchen use. Agave is available as a light (filtered) or dark syrup. Luo han guo is available as a powdered fruit extract.

**Special Considerations:** Stevia and luo han guo are hundreds of times sweeter than common sugar and should be used sparingly. Xylitol does not break down completely in the intestines, and large amounts may cause diarrhea.

# 12

# Omega-3 Essential Fatty Acids

Fat has a bad reputation—many people associate dietary fat with obesity, heart disease and other chronic conditions. But not all fat is bad fat. Some fats, known as omega-3 fatty acids, can lower the risk of heart disease, fight arthritis and other inflammatory diseases, improve brain function and enhance immune function.

In the late 1970s, Danish researchers compared the rates of heart disease among Eskimos in Greenland to those among Danish populations. Despite their high-fat diet, the Eskimos were much less likely to suffer from heart disease than their Danish counterparts. How could this be?

Scientists hypothesized that Eskimos experienced such low rates of heart disease because of their consumption of fish, whales and other marine mammals, all of which are high in omega-3 polyunsaturated fatty acids. Epidemiological studies of fish-eating populations in Japan and elsewhere supported this hypothesis, and subsequent research confirmed it. In 2000, researchers at the Mid America Heart Institute in Kansas City wrote that more than 4,500 studies confirmed the cardiovascular benefits of omega-3 fatty acids. The research on omega-3 fatty acids from marine sources may also apply to omega-3 fatty acids from flaxseed and other plant sources.

# Not All Fats Are Created Equal

The human body can produce most of the fat it needs from carbon, hydrogen and oxygen. But the body can't produce omega-3 and omega-6 fatty acids, although it needs both. Because these fats must be obtained from the diet, they are called essential fatty acids, or EFAs.

## TYPES OF EFA SUPPLEMENTS

Essential fatty acids, especially fish oil products, are sold under a variety of names. They may be called fish oil, omega-3 fatty acids or EFAs, or they may be called by specific oil names such as DHA or EPA. Most fish oil products contain a mixture of DHA and EPA, no matter what they're called. When in doubt, simply read the ingredient label.

Flaxseed products are available as liquids and in gelatin capsules. Flaxseed oil is sometimes sold by itself and sometimes mixed with other omega-3 fatty acids. Again, when in doubt, check the label.

There are three types of omega-3 fatty acids: eicosapentaenoic acid (EPA), docosahexaenoic acid (DHA) and alpha-linolenic acid (ALA). The body can most readily use EPA and DHA, which are found primarily in fish and marine mammals. The body converts ALA, which comes from plant sources such as flaxseed, into DHA and EPA.

The other essential fatty acids—omega-6 fatty acids—are vital to our health, but most of us get too much of them in our diet. Most vegetable oils today are high in omega-6 fatty acids and low in omega-3 fatty acids, and the imbalance can cause health problems like heart disease, cancer and autoimmune disease.

For instance, a 2004 article in the *New England Journal of Medicine* linked cystic fibrosis to an imbalance of fatty acids.

In today's diets, the ratio of omega-6 to omega-3 fatty acids is nearly 15 to one—far from the ideal one-to-one ratio of essential fatty acids that scientists believe our ancestors ate. However, we can probably improve our overall health even without achieving the ideal ratio. In 2002, Artemis Simopoulos, president of the Center for Genetics, Nutrition and Health in Washington, DC, reported that the EFA ratio needed to reduce health risks varies from condition to condition. For example, a four-to-one omega-6 to omega-3 ratio may reduce the risk of dying from heart disease by 70 percent, but reducing the spread of colon cancer requires a 2.5-to-one ratio.

# How Do Essential Fats Help the Body?

EFAs can help reduce the stickiness of blood platelets, reducing the risk of atherosclerosis (hardening of the arteries), stroke and heart attack. EFAs can also help lower levels of triglycerides and LDL cholesterol. EFAs have even been shown to have anti-inflammatory effects that can help fight illnesses such as arthritis, irritable bowel syndrome, asthma and more. In fact, EFAs in breast milk may reduce the risks of asthma and other atopic conditions in children.

# Health Benefits of EFAs

## Cardiovascular Health

Research shows that omega-3 fats can lower blood pressure, decrease LDL ("bad") cholesterol levels, increase HDL ("good") cholesterol levels and reduce the risk of heart attack, stroke and other vascular disorders. When heart attacks do happen, omega-3 fatty acids may make them less severe.

Omega-3s reduce the risk or severity of heart disease by influencing several factors, including blood clotting and blood pressure. There is also mounting evidence that omega-3s can protect the heart against arrhythmias (irregular heart rhythms), which can be fatal. According to the American Heart Association, arrhythmias are responsible for more than 780,000 hospitalizations per year.

In August 2003, an article in the *European Journal of Medical Research* reported that omega-3 fatty acid could reduce the risk of sudden cardiac death in as little as 90 days. The fatty acids were reported to be as effective as aspirin and statins in reducing the risk of sudden death from heart disease. The only treatment that proved more effective than omega-3 fatty acids was the use of beta-blockers, but even patients taking beta-blockers benefited from the addition of omega-3 fatty acids.

In 2004, the FDA recognized the health benefits of EFAs by approving a qualified health claim for products containing omega-3 fatty acids. Food and supplement companies can now state on the product label that EPA and DHA fatty acids may reduce the risk of coronary heart disease (CHD).

Also in 2004, a team of researchers wrote an article in *Preventive Medicine* proposing the "Omega-3 Index," which they defined as the red blood cell composition of EPA and DHA. According to the authors, the Omega-3 Index is a reflection of long-term omega-3 intake and is a simple indicator of CHD risk.

## Arthritis

Most studies on the antiarthritic effects of EFAs focus on the effects of omega-3 fatty acids on rheumatoid arthritis. Rheumatoid arthritis is an autoimmune disorder in which the immune system attacks the joints, causing pain and stiffness. In 1995, a meta-analysis in the *Journal of Clinical Epidemiology* revealed that taking fish oil supplements for at least three months resulted in modest but significant improvement in joint tenderness and morning stiffness. In 1996, a population-based study published in *Epidemiology* suggested that omega-3 fatty acids help prevent rheumatoid arthritis. The study's authors reported that women who ate two or more servings of broiled or baked fish per week had about half the risk of developing rheumatoid arthritis as women who ate less than one serving per week.

## Cancer and Other Conditions

Research indicates that omega-3 fatty acids may help prevent and treat certain cancers. A meta-analysis published in 2007 in the *American Journal of Epidemiology* reported that fish consumption could provide a slight reduction in colorectal cancer risk. The same year, researchers from the Oregon Health and Science University conducted a large-scale study on fatty acids and breast cancer in Shanghai, China. They found that omega-3 fatty acids provided a protective effect against breast cancer. Also in 2007, researchers from Wake Forest University in North Carolina investigated the effects of fatty acids on prostate cancer risk in genetically predisposed mice and found that omega-3 fatty acids reduced prostate tumor growth, while omega-6 fatty acids did the opposite.

There are other uses for omega-3 fatty acids. Researchers are looking into the links between fish oil and childhood asthma, healthier pregnancies (and healthier infants), improved bone growth, schizophrenia, Alzheimer's disease and lengthened remission time for patients in prolonged remission from Crohn's disease. Some experts also believe that essential fatty acids can help lower the risk and severity of depression.

# Where to Find Omega-3 Fatty Acids

Fish—especially fatty fish—is an excellent source of EPA and DHA, and the American Heart Association recommends eating at least two servings weekly. However, some fish, especially larger, predatory species, may contain mercury, PCBs and other harmful toxins that can cause serious health problems.

Vegetarian sources of omega-3 fatty acids such as walnuts, soybeans and flaxseed are free of such toxins. These sources provide omega-3 fatty acids such as ALA, which the body must convert into EPA and DHA. The extent to which ALA is converted to EPA and DHA is still undetermined.

Supplements may be the best option for those who wish to ensure safe, optimal intake of omega-3 fatty acids. Fish oil supplements provide high levels of EPA and DHA and are generally free from mercury and PCBs. Krill oil, a newcomer to the supplement scene, is also an excellent choice. In addition to omega-3 fatty acids, krill oil contains astaxanthin, a potent carotenoid antioxidant. Plus, krill oil is free of the fishy aftertaste associated with fish oil. For people who want vegetarian EFAs, flaxseed oil is a rich source of ALA.

# The Bottom Line

Omega-3 fatty acids provide the body with vital building blocks that affect nearly every body system. From preventing cancer to battling arthritis to promoting heart health, these essential fats can do wonders for disease prevention and treatment. Fish oil and flaxseed oil are associated with a wide range of scientifically confirmed health benefits, making them some of today's most valuable and popular dietary supplements.

## OMEGA-3 FAST FACTS

The Three Types of Omega-3 Essential fatty acids include: EPA (eicosapentaenoic acid), DHA (docosahexaenoic acid), and ALA (alpha-linolenic acid).

**Uses and Benefits:** Omega-3 fatty acids may benefit people with angina, arthritis, asthma, breast cancer, colon cancer, constipation, dermatitis, gout, heart disease, high blood pressure, high cholesterol, inflammatory conditions, irritable bowel syndrome, lupus, migraines, mood disorders, multiple sclerosis, osteoarthritis, rheumatoid arthritis, sciatica, stroke and suppressed immunity.

**Sources:** Dietary sources of EFAs include fatty fish (such as albacore, bluefish, herring, mackerel, rainbow trout, salmon), walnuts, flaxseed, soybeans and canola oil. EFA supplements include fish oil, flaxseed oil and krill oil.

**Special Considerations:** Because of their blood-thinning capabilities, omega-3 fatty acids may increase bleeding time, leading to more frequent nosebleeds and easy bruising. Do not take EFAs if you have a bleeding disorder, if you are on anticoagulants or if you are allergic to fish. Diabetics should consult with their physician before using EFAs. Flaxseed is generally regarded as safe.

# 13

# Probiotics

The word *bacteria* may invoke images of something harmful or unsanitary—spoiled food, perhaps, or a dirty bathroom. However, many bacteria are beneficial to our health. Our bodies are teeming with trillions of bacteria from numerous species that promote healthy digestion, produce vitamins, fight infection and enhance immune function, among other things. To put this into perspective, each person's digestive tract contains between three and four *pounds* of beneficial bacteria, or *probiotics*. Two particular types of bacteria—*Lactobacillus acidophilus* (often called acidophilus) and *Bifidobacterium bifidum*—are among the most helpful of these probiotics.

## Battle for the Gut

We are not born with a ready-made supply of beneficial bacteria, but we begin to acquire them soon after birth. Initially, infants receive beneficial bacteria from their mother's breast milk. As infants grow and start to eat other types of food, additional bacteria—both good and bad—begin to colonize their bodies. As we mature, an ongoing battle rages as beneficial bacteria and harmful microbes fight for domination of the gut and other parts of the body. By maintaining optimal levels of beneficial bacteria, we can keep the harmful varieties in check, thereby preventing a host of gastrointestinal maladies and keeping a variety of diseases at bay.

# The Good, the Bad, and the Ugly

A strong population of beneficial bacteria in the gut largely neutralizes any unwelcome intruders that enter the body, such as molds, yeasts and harmful bacteria. When the gastrointestinal tract is thoroughly colonized by beneficial bacteria, harmful pathogens will find no suitable place to form new colonies. Conversely, if harmful bacteria dominate the gut, they will welcome more of their kind and fend off beneficial bacteria, creating an ugly pathogen- and toxin-ridden digestive tract that can create serious health problems throughout the body. This condition is called dysbiosis.

# Antibiotics Kill Beneficial Bacteria, Too

Ironically, one of the greatest threats to beneficial bacteria is something that is used to treat illness and promote health—antibiotics. While antibiotics serve a critical, and sometimes life-saving, function in treating infections caused by harmful bacteria, they also decimate the body's colonies of beneficial bacteria. This decrease in beneficial bacteria sets the stage for pathogen proliferation in the gut, secondary infection and, eventually, resistance to antibiotics themselves.

## Antibiotics and Vaginal Yeast Infections

One example of the detrimental effects of antibiotics on the delicate balance of natural flora involves the proliferation of vaginal yeast infections in women who take antibiotics.

Vaginal yeast is held in check by acidophilus and other beneficial bacteria. Once an antibiotic kills those bacteria, the yeast multiply and spread quickly, causing a yeast infection. Symptoms of yeast infections include itching, burning, redness, irritation and painful sexual intercourse. Chronic yeast infections are an increasingly common health problem among women; if left untreated, they can lead to more serious health conditions.

Acute yeast infections can be safely and effectively treated with over-the-counter medications, but these remedies don't offer long-term solutions to avoiding chronic infections. Probiotic supplements and dairy products that contain living bacterial cultures (such as yogurt and kefir) do. By helping to reestablish colonies of *B. bifidum*, *L. acidophilus* and other beneficial bacteria, these foods and supplements help maintain a healthy microbial balance in the vagina and surrounding tissues.

## Conditions that can result from an unhealthy imbalance of intestinal bacteria

Acne
Allergies
Arthritis
Asthma
Attention deficit disorder
Candida
Chronic fatigue
Colitis
Constipation
Crohn's disease
Depression
Diarrhea

Eczema and psoriasis
Endometriosis
Fibromyalgia
Gastritis
Headaches
Hormonal disturbances
Hypoglycemia
Irritable bowel disease
Menstrual disorders
Obesity
Vaginal infections

# Other Enemies to Beneficial Bacteria

Antibiotics are not the only threat to beneficial bacteria. Other factors that can deplete beneficial bacteria levels include poor diet, stress, disease, food allergies and sensitivities, high levels of toxins, too much sugar or refined carbohydrates, alcohol abuse and tobacco use. When attempting to restore a healthy balance of intestinal flora, consider how these factors apply to you and take action to address them. Manage stress, cut back on refined carbohydrates and get tested for food allergies. Even simple changes can have a profound effect on your gastrointestinal health and overall well-being.

# Which Bacteria Are Most Beneficial?

Hundreds of species of bacteria inhabit the body, but only a handful of these species are beneficial. The following probiotics offer you the most health benefits.

*Lactobacillus acidophilus.* Out of about 200 strains of acidophilus, the most beneficial are the NAS and DDS-1 strains. Both protect against the pathogens *Bacillus subtilis, Serratia marcescens, Proteus vulgaris, Pseudomonas fluorescens, Pseudomonas aeruginosa, Escherichia coli, Sarcina lutea, Staphylococcus aureus*, and *Streptococcus lactis*. The NAS and DDS-1 strains of acidophilus have also been shown to inhibit fungal growth, relieve chronic constipation and diarrhea, increase the production of lactase and improve the absorption of nutrients (especially calcium). Other lactobacillus strains that can benefit intestinal health include *Lactobacillus rhamnosus, Lactobacillus casei* and *Lactobacillus johnsonii*.

***Bifidobacterium bifidum.*** This important probiotic inhabits the large intestine of adults and aggressively destroys pathogens. *B. bifidum* helps produce B vitamins and inhibits the bacteria that convert nitrates into cancer-causing nitrites. Interestingly, *B. bifidum* may be most beneficial for those whom acidophilus supplements don't help. Many experts consider *B. bifidum* to be preferable to acidophilus for children and adults with liver disorders.

Additionally, a growing body of research indicates that the "superstrain" *B. bifidum* Malyoth offers widespread health benefits, detoxifying the liver, preventing nutrient malabsorption and B-vitamin deficiencies, regulating waste production and preventing diarrhea and constipation.

***Lactobacillus bulgaricus.*** *L. bulgaricus* plays a supporting role, helping other probiotics effectively colonize the gut. One of the most notable strains of *L. bulgaricus*, LB-51, has received praise for its ability to treat a range of digestive problems. LB-51 has also proven to be effective in destroying harmful bacteria and stimulating immune response. Research also indicates that LB-51 helps to maintain a clean intestinal tract, thus alleviating constipation and diarrhea.

***Lactobacillus GG.*** Many experts believe that *Lactobacillus GG* (LGG) is superior to *L. acidophilus* in its ability to fight gastrointestinal disorders. In fact, the beneficial attributes of LGG have more scientific support than those of acidophilus and other probiotics. One reason may be that LGG is derived from the sterile form of a bacteria that grows in the human intestine, whereas acidophilus comes from a bovine source. Because of its human origin, LGG may be better equipped to survive in the gastrointestinal tract and vagina.

# Selecting High-Quality Living Probiotic Supplements

Many high-quality probiotic supplements are available today, but there's one overarching consideration when selecting a supplement: probiotics are *living* organisms, and if they are to have any therapeutic value, they must be alive when you ingest them.

Probiotics are available in several different forms, including powder, capsule, tablet, wafer and liquid. Experts tend to prefer powders and capsules, especially enteric-coated capsules, which pass through the stomach intact and release the bacteria directly into the intestinal tract. Some experts discourage the use of liquid probiotics, as they can lose their potency fairly quickly.

Most experts recommend looking for supplements with at least one billion organisms per capsule or two billion organisms per teaspoon. Some products offer even more.

Whichever product you choose, ensure that it has a guaranteed expiration date. If it doesn't, don't buy it. Also, beware of products that qualify potencies with statements like "at the time of manufacture" or "at the time of shipment." Who knows how long after those dates you will actually buy the product!

Avoid products that indicate they have undergone a centrifuge or ultrafiltration process. These processes can break down the bacteria, rendering them less effective or even useless. They also artificially inflate the bacterial count by including damaged and partial organisms in the count.

Store probiotics in a cool, dry place, and keep the lid on tight. The refrigerator is a great place to keep probiotic supplements, but be careful they don't freeze.

Take probiotics on an empty stomach first thing in the morning, and then close to mealtimes throughout the day. Some experts recommend taking probiotics with filtered, lukewarm water because tap water may contain chlorine, which will kill bacteria, and cold water can have a debilitating effect on bacteria.

Don't take probiotics and antibiotics at the same time; the antibiotics will simply kill the probiotics, rendering them useless. Some experts recommend doubling or even tripling your normal probiotic dose for three weeks after finishing antibiotic treatment.

## The Bottom Line

Decades of research indicate that friendly bacteria offer wide-ranging benefits for you and your health. They defend against dangerous pathogens, including harmful bacteria, fungi and yeast such as *Candida albicans*. Probiotics also help produce vital nutrients and digestive enzymes. They discourage infections of the vagina and urinary tract, prevent diarrhea and constipation, alleviate various gastrointestinal ills, lower high cholesterol and can even relieve symptoms of lupus and fibromyalgia.

## PROBIOTIC FAST FACTS

**Popular Strains:** *Lactobacillus acidophilus*, *Lactobacillus bulgaricus*, *Bifidobacterium bifidum*, *Lactobacillus GG*.

**Uses and Benefits:** Probiotics may benefit people with chronic yeast infections, urinary tract infections, lactose intolerance, diarrhea, constipation, impaired immune response, irritable bowel syndrome, lupus, fibromyalgia, high cholesterol, indigestion, nutrient malabsorption, bloating, gas, osteoporosis and B-vitamin deficiencies.

**Sources:** Dietary sources of probiotics include fermented milk products (such as yogurt and kefir), kimchi, kombucha tea, sauerkraut, soy sauce, tempeh, miso and pickled vegetables. Probiotics supplements are available as powders, capsules, tablets, wafers and liquids (experts generally prefer powders and enteric-coated capsules).

**Special Considerations:** Probiotic supplements are quite safe. However, some reports indicate that taking more than ten billion viable organisms daily may cause mild gastrointestinal distress. If you suffer from a severe gastrointestinal problem such as pancreatic disease, consult with your health-care provider before taking probiotics

# 14

# Soy

Soy is one of the world's largest and most important food crops. Because of their complete amino acid profile, soybeans can provide as much protein as meat, milk and other animal foods. Ounce for ounce, soybeans provide more protein than beef, more calcium than milk and more lecithin than eggs. Because 35 to 38 percent of the calories in soybeans are derived from protein, the World Health Organization has assigned soy foods the highest possible score for protein content.

Soybeans are rich in chemical compounds called phytochemicals, which may help prevent disease and promote overall health and wellness. Two particular phytochemicals in soybeans—dadzein and genistein—are powerful antioxidants. Other phytochemicals in soy can help lower cholesterol levels, reduce the risk of heart disease, protect against cancer and provide support for healthy immune function. Soy foods are also excellent sources of potassium, zinc and most B vitamins.

# Soy Foods

While soybeans have an outstanding nutritional profile, few people would just sit down and eat a bowl of freshly picked soybeans. Soybeans are almost always served cooked, and most of the soy foods that people eat today require a considerable amount of processing. The following are some popular soy foods:

## Soy Milk

Soy milk is made by grinding soybeans and mixing them with water. Many flavors and types of soy milk are readily available. Because it can be used in many of the same ways as dairy milk, soy milk has become a popular alternative to dairy products in the United States.

## Tofu

Tofu is a brick of soy curd made by pureeing cooked soybeans and forming them into white custard-like cakes. Tofu has little flavor of its own and can be a used in a multitude of other dishes. Tofu is available in silken, soft and firm textures. Silken tofu can be used to make smoothies and sauces, and firm tofu works well in stir-fries.

## Natto

Natto is a somewhat stinky fermented soy food made by incubating cooked soybeans in straw. The straw contains the bacterium *Bacillus natto*, which aids in the fermentation process. Natto is eaten as a breakfast food in parts of Japan, and recent studies have shown that natto offers important cardioprotective qualities. In the United States, natto is usually available from Asian specialty grocers.

## Tempeh

Tempeh is made by pressing cooked whole soybeans into a dense cake that can be cut into pieces and used in various recipes. Because of its rich flavor and chewy texture, tempeh is an excellent meat substitute for vegetarians.

## Miso

Miso is a fermented soybean paste that can be used to flavor soups and a variety of other dishes.

## Soy Sauce

Widely used in Asian cooking, soy sauce is a fermented blend of cooked soybeans, grain and salty brine.

## Soy Protein Powder

Soy is available in a wide range of protein powder supplements that can be used to make smoothies and other tasty beverages. These protein powders are a cost-effective way to add soy protein to your diet.

# Soy and Women's Health

Soy contains phytoestrogens called isoflavones. Phytoestrogens are naturally occurring plant compounds that mimic natural estrogens. Because of their isoflavone content, soy products can play an important role in women's health, providing relief from the symptoms of premenstrual syndrome, easing symptoms of menopause, and preventing hormone-induced cancers.

## Premenstrual Syndrome

Many women suffering from the monthly effects of premenstrual syndrome (PMS) have benefited from incorporating soy and soy supplements into their diet. PMS manifests itself to varying degrees through symptoms such as acne, bloating, backache, fatigue, extreme irritability, headache, sore or swollen breasts and depression. Several studies have shown that soy foods and soy supplements can have a beneficial impact on the effects of PMS. In short, soy isoflavones occupy estrogen receptor sites, causing a decrease in circulating estrogen. Lower levels of estrogen are known to result in fewer or less severe symptoms of PMS.

## Menopause

Soy protein is marketed as an alternative to hormone replacement therapy for women going through menopause. Soy isoflavones bind to the body's estrogen receptors, but they are much weaker than the human hormone, so they probably do not increase the risk of hormone-induced cancers such as breast cancer. For women who cannot or do not want to receive estrogen replacement therapy, soy supplements may provide adequate relief from hot flashes and other menopausal symptoms.

## Cancer

The prospect of developing hormone-induced cancers (like breast cancer and ovarian cancer) is a major concern among middle-aged and older women. Fortunately, soy isoflavones such as genistein have shown impressive results in fighting cancer.

Genistein, which has only about one one-thousandth the hormone potency of estrogen, attaches to estrogen receptor sites in breast cells, preventing the much more potent and potentially carcinogenic estrogen from attaching to these same receptor sites.

Genistein also helps prevent cancer by slowing the activity of the hypothalamus and pituitary gland, which both contribute to estrogen production in the ovaries. When less estrogen flows through a woman's body, her cycle lasts longer, translating to fewer cycles over her lifetime. Ultimately, this means that her exposure to estrogen will be less, thereby decreasing her risk of breast cancer and other conditions.

Researchers believe that genistein helps control tumor growth by enhancing apoptosis, or programmed cell death, which regulates all cell growth by not allowing them to reproduce too quickly.

Studies have also shown that genistein and other isoflavones can inhibit angiogenesis, the process by which new blood vessels are formed to feed tumors. Stopping this process causes tumors to become nutrient-starved and shrink.

There is also some indication that genistein may help the mammary gland cells to mature and diversify, thereby cutting the risk of cancer. The mammary glands of women who have never nursed are more immature and thereby more vulnerable to cancer formation.

# Other Health Benefits of Soy

## *Antioxidant*

The antioxidant properties of isoflavones may help LDL ("bad") cholesterol resist oxidation and prevent free radical damage to DNA. Antioxidants may also defend against cancer. Studies show that genestein has greater antioxidant activities than the other isoflavones. Genestein may also increase the production of antioxidant enzymes, such as superoxide dismutase.

## Bone Health

Researchers around the world are excited about soy's ability to strengthen bones, increase bone mass and prevent osteoporosis. Soy is a great dietary source of calcium, and calcium is essential for healthy bones and proper development of the musculoskeletal system. Additionally, genistein and daidzein appear to inhibit the breakdown of bones. One study showed that soy isoflavones helped fortify bones found in the lumbar spine and also prevented the development of dowager's hump, which is commonly seen in postmenopausal women. Another study showed that genistein was equal to prescription doses of estradiol for retaining bone mineral mass.

## Heart Health

Numerous studies have shown that soy and soy isoflavones can benefit the cardiovascular system in many ways. And so impressive are its heart-healthy attributes that in 2000, the FDA allowed soy food products to carry a health claim stating that soy is effective in fighting coronary heart disease. While results have been mixed, there is promising research surrounding both genistein and daidzein and their complementary effect in fighting heart disease.

## Reducing Cholesterol Levels

It is well established in controlled trials that increased soy protein intake has the potential to lower LDL-cholesterol levels and thus may also reduce the risk of heart disease, particularly in postmenopausal women.

# Even More Health Benefits

Aside from the benefits surrounding hormone-related conditions in women, heart disease and cancer, soy and its principal components are showing promise in helping other areas, including the following:

- Fighting bacterial and fungal infections
- Acting as a diuretic
- Improving kidney function
- Relieving effects of type 2 diabetes
- Preventing gallstones

# The Bottom Line

Soy is a nutritious, affordable and widely available source of complete protein. The fact that soy may provide so many more health benefits is all the more reason to add soy to your daily diet.

---

### SOY FAST FACTS

**Uses and Benefits:** Soy is a natural, meat-free source of complete protein. Soy may also provide nutritive support for women's health and cardiovascular health.

**Sources:** Soy foods include tofu, soy milk, natto, tempeh, miso and soy sauce. Soy protein powder is widely available, as are supplements containing soy extracts.

**Special Considerations:** Soy and soy foods are widely considered to be safe. However in some cases soy isoflavones have been reported to impair thyroid activity. Discuss any concerns you may have with your physician before increasing the amount of soy in your diet.

# 15

# Superfruits

Everyone should eat a wide variety of fruits and vegetables. Scientific evidence reveals that fruits and vegetables, which are rich sources of vitamins, minerals, antioxidants and other phytonutrients, can help prevent disease and boost overall health. Recently, several novel fruits have gained popularity throughout America for their incredible nutritional value. These "superfruits" include açaí berry, mangosteen, goji berry and the more familiar pomegranate.

## **Açaí Berry**

The açaí berry is a small purple fruit that is as great tasting as it is healthy, thanks to its high content of powerful antioxidants. Açaí is native to the swamps and floodplains of Central and South America, but today açaí products—capsules, powders, juices and more—are readily available from health food stores, Web sites and even warehouse clubs.

The main sources of antioxidants in açaí are anthocyanins, the pigments that give the berries their purple color. Açaí contains 10 to 33 times the amount of anthocyanins found in red wine, which researchers have studied for its role in preventing heart disease. Açaí is more than a source of antioxidants—the berry also contains amino acids, unsaturated fats and phytosterols, all of which promote health throughout the entire body.

# Nutritional Benefits of Açaí

## *Phytosterols*

Açaí contains beta-sitosterol and other valuable phytosterols. Phytosterols, also referred to as plant sterols, are natural substances with chemical structures similar to that of cholesterol. Phytosterols are found in plant cells and membranes and provide numerous benefits to the human body: they reduce harmful cholesterol levels; they may support immune system health; they may even be an effective treatment for benign prostate hyperplasia, a common condition among middle-aged and elderly men.

## *Other Nutrients*

Açaí is rich in calcium, vitamins C and E, unsaturated fats, iron, manganese, chromium, copper and boron. The açaí berry is so rich in nutrients, it could almost be considered a multivitamin in the form of a fruit!

# Açaí and Your Health

Açaí's abundant nutrients have important effects on your health.

## Fiber for Digestive Support and Cancer Prevention

Açaí is an excellent source of fiber. Research demonstrates that a high-fiber diet can help protect against cancer, diabetes, heart disease and obesity. Many people only get about half the fiber they need each day, but adding açaí and other fruits and vegetables to the diet can help fill that gap.

## Anti-Inflammatory Properties

Many health experts believe that inflammation, which occurs as a result of disease, injuries and autoimmune disorders (when the body attacks its own tissues), may contribute to the development of some chronic diseases. Açaí contains powerful antioxidants that help alleviate inflammation by neutralizing enzymes that attack connective tissues.

## Protection for Blood Vessels

Free radicals damage the endothelial cells that line blood vessel walls. This damage eventually leads to a buildup of arterial plaque, which can lead to atherosclerosis and heart disease. By protecting endothelial cells from free radicals, the anthocyanins in açaí support blood vessel health and protect against cardiovascular disease.

## Effects of Diabetes

Diabetic retinopathy is a severe complication of diabetes in which elevated blood sugar levels damage blood vessels in the retina, the light-sensitive tissue in the eye. Severe cases of retinopathy may cause blindness; in fact, diabetic retinopathy is the leading cause of blindness in American adults. Anthocyanins protect against this capillary damage by preventing free radical damage to the circulatory system.

# **Mangosteen**

The mangosteen is a small purple fruit, roughly the size and shape of a medium tomato, that grows throughout Southeast Asia. Slicing open a mangosteen reveals a deep red rind, called the pericarp, about half an inch thick, which protects the white segmented flesh and the black seeds at the fruit's heart. It is the pericarp, dried and powdered, that has been used in traditional medicine systems throughout Singapore, India and China.

The deep red color of the mangosteen's pericarp indicates its rich content of polyphenolic antioxidants such as catechins and tannins. Unfortunately, these antioxidants are extremely astringent, and their high concentration makes the pericarp practically inedible. Although the pectin-rich pericarp has been made into an edible jelly in some countries, it must first be soaked in a 6 percent brine solution to reduce its astringency and increase its palatability. In addition to polyphenols, the pericarp contains xanthones, phenolic plant compounds that may have antitumor, antibacterial and fungicidal properties.

# Nutritional Benefits of Mangosteen

## *Catechins*

Mangosteen pericarp is extremely rich in catechins. Catechins are polyphenols, phytochemicals with significant antioxidant activity. Catechins are related to tannins, the chemicals that cause your mouth to pucker when eating unripe fruit, and have found their claim to fame in green tea. They are also found in abundance in grapes, wine and chocolate. In addition their antioxidant ability, catechins are known for their potential to reduce body fat, and the National Cancer

Institute reports that catechins may even help prevent cancer. An average mangosteen pericarp contains 50 to 60 milligrams of catechins, the same amount found in 100 grams of dark chocolate.

## Xanthones: Promising Superheroes

Like catechins, xanthones are polyphenols. Mangosteen pericarp is rich in mangostin, a xanthone with antibacterial, fungicidal and antitumor properties. In 1995, researchers at the University of Western Australia showed that mangostin can inhibit the oxidation of LDL cholesterol, which is implicated in plaque formation in atherosclerosis.

# Mangosteen and Your Health

## Cancer Research

Research suggests that mangosteen may someday play a role in cancer treatment and prevention. In 2002, the journal *Planta Medica* published the results of a study in which researchers in Taipei, Taiwan, studied the effects of six mangosteen-derived xanthones on human cancer cells. The researchers reported that a xanthone derivative called garcinone E killed lung, liver and gastric cancer cells. In 2004, Japanese researchers reported that mangostin derived from mangosteen pericarp induced apoptosis (cell death) in leukemia cells.

## Antibacterial Properties

In 1996, Japanese researchers conducted an in vitro study on the antibacterial activity of xanthones and found that xanthones inhibited antibiotic-resistant strains of the *Staphylococcus aureus* bacteria, the most common cause of staph infections. The results of this study were published in the August 1996 issue of the *Journal of Pharmacy and Pharmacology*. According to another in vitro study, published in July 2003 in the *Chemical & Pharmaceutical Bulletin*, xanthones from mangosteen may inhibit the bacteria responsible for tuberculosis.

# **Goji Berry**

The power of the goji berry is no secret in China, where the berry has been used for its many healing properties for thousands of years. According to the *Ben Cao Gang Mu*, a well-known Chinese herbal compiled in the late sixteenth century, "Taking in Chinese goji berry regularly may regulate the flow of vital energy and strengthen the physique, which can lead to longevity." Recently, the goji berry has been discovered in the West, and its amazing antioxidant and health benefits are now available to all.

## *Modern Uses of the Goji Berry*

Building on ancient knowledge of the goji berry, modern scientists have extensively researched the fruit's nutritional profile and health-promoting properties. Studies provide evidence that the goji berry fights free radicals, supports a healthy immune system, improves vision and maintains healthy blood sugar levels.

The Chinese Ministry of Public Health approved sales of the goji berry as a botanical medicine in 1983, and the Chinese State Scientific and Technological commission has declared the goji berry a national treasure.

# Nutritional Benefits of the Goji Berry

According to a study conducted by the Beijing National Research Institute in 1988, goji berries contain 21 trace minerals, 18 amino acids, over 500 times more vitamin C than oranges, more beta-carotene than carrots and more calcium than spinach. An eight-ounce portion of goji berries contains 4,000 percent of the RDI (Reference Daily Intake) for vitamin B1, 1,000 percent of the RDI for vitamin B3, 190 percent of the RDI for fiber and over 100 percent of the RDI for chromium.

In addition, goji berries are full of flavonoids, the water-soluble pigments that give blueberries, peppers and oranges their vivid colors. Flavonoids are also powerful antioxidants. In January 2009, a team of researchers in Phoenix, Arizona, reported that regular consumption of goji berries could increase antioxidant markers in humans. According to the results of their double-blind, placebo-controlled trial, subjects who consumed 120 milliliters of goji juice per day for 30 days experienced a significant increase in three antioxidant markers.

# Goji Berries and Your Health

## *Healthy Immune System Support*

Goji berries provide support for a healthy immune system. Thus far, most studies on the effects of goji berries on immunity have focused on mice. However, in 2003 researchers from the Huazhong University of Science and Technology in China reported that a goji compound could be used to induce an immune response in human cells. Specifically, the researchers found that goji stimulated interleukin 2 and tumor growth necrosis factor—two compounds essential for the immune response to cancer.

## *Improved Vision*

Both ancient tradition and modern research suggest that goji berries can improve vision. Lutein and zeaxanthin, two pigments contained in goji berries, protect the retina by neutralizing the free radicals from sunlight. Chinese researchers tested the effects of goji berries on the eyesight of 27 subjects and reported positive results: dark adaptation dramatically improved; physiologic scotomas (blind spots) decreased; and serum vitamin A and carotene content—indicators of eyesight acuity—increased.

## Healthy Blood Sugar and Cholesterol Levels

The goji berry may support blood sugar and cholesterol levels, helping to prevent diabetes, pre-diabetic conditions and cardiovascular disease.

Researchers at the University of Hong Kong and Wuhan University conducted a study of the glucose-stabilizing properties of the goji berry. According to their report, "It was found that the three *Lycium barbarum* [goji berry] fruit extracts/fractions could significantly reduce blood glucose levels and serum total cholesterol (TC) and triglyceride (TG) concentrations and at the same time markedly increase high density lipoprotein cholesterol (HDL-c) levels after ten days treatment in tested rabbits, indicating that there were substantial hypoglycemic and hypolipidemic effects." In other words, their research revealed that goji berries decreased the amount of blood sugar and total cholesterol in the blood while increasing the amount of "good" HDL cholesterol.

# **Pomegranate**

Pomegranates have been grown in the Middle East since ancient times. They have also been cultivated in the Mediterranean region, Europe, Asia, Africa and India. The pomegranate tree was introduced to California in the late eighteenth century; today, pomegranates in the United States are grown primarily in Arizona and California.

Pomegranates are basically round with a tough reddish-pink skin. Cutting the fruit open reveals white, fleshy tissue and hundreds of pips—small translucent sacs that contain juice, tart red pulp and a seed. To eat a pomegranate, slice it in half and place it in a bowl of water. Gently remove the pips from the rind and membrane and strain the pips from the water. Then, enjoy the tart, rich flavor of the pips by themselves, or use them on salads and in baked goods.

## Nutritional Benefits of Pomegranate

Pomegranates are an excellent source of potassium, vitamin C and polyphenols, especially anthocyanins, ellagic acid, tannins and punicalagin (of all the polyphenols contained in pomegranate juice, punicalagin is responsible for half of the juice's antioxidant power). In one study, researchers compared pomegranate juice with cranberry juice, red wine, blueberry juice and orange juice and found that pomegranate juice had more polyphenols than the other juices and that the polyphenols in pomegranate juice were significantly more active. Pomegranate juice neutralized free radicals and prevented LDL cholesterol oxidation, which contributes to atherosclerosis.

## Pomegranate and Your Health

Scientific literature increasingly shows that the polyphenols in pomegranate juice protect the heart, fight free radicals and protect against cancer and other chronic diseases.

Studies suggest that regularly drinking pomegranate juice helps to reduce oxidative stress, atherosclerosis, blood pressure and narrowing of the carotid arteries in the neck. Scientists at the Preventive Medicine Research Center in Sausalito, California, found that 240 milliliters (about eight ounces) of pomegranate juice a day improved blood flow to the heart in patients with coronary heart disease.

In 2006, Israeli researchers reported that the antioxidants in pomegranate juice are especially beneficial for diabetics. Noting that diabetes increases oxidative stress and the risk of atherosclerosis, the researchers gave 10 diabetic patients 50 milliliters of pomegranate juice per day for three months. (As a control, 10 non-diabetic patients received the same amount of pomegranate juice.) The researchers found that pomegranate juice reduced the risk of oxidation and atherosclerosis in the diabetic patients without increasing blood sugar levels.

Pomegranate juice may even protect against cancer. Laboratory and animal studies have revealed potential roles for pomegranate in fighting lung cancer, skin cancer, prostate cancer, colon cancer and breast cancer.

## The Bottom Line

As baby boomers reach their fifties and sixties, the emphasis on active lifestyles, maintaining good health and living longer increases. To meet their health goals, more and more people are turning to fruits and vegetables for the healthful antioxidants they contain. As modern science continues to research the role of free-radical damage in aging and disease, expect to hear more about the potent phytochemicals in açaí berries, mangosteen, goji berries and pomegranate, all of which offer numerous benefits to those who want to take control of their health.

## SUPERFRUITS FAST FACTS

**Uses and Benefits:** Superfruits are nutritional powerhouses, providing vitamins, minerals, antioxidants, phytonutrients and more. Because of their nutritional value, superfruits may boost overall well-being and help prevent disease.

**Forms:** Superfruits are whole foods and can be enjoyed as such. Many are also available as juices or fruit extracts. Because of its astringency, the highly nutritious mangosteen pericarp is inedible—look for supplements instead.

# 16

# Turmeric

What do Worcestershire sauce, mustard and Middle Eastern cuisine have in common? All feature turmeric, the yellow, peppery spice commonly associated with Indian curries. And new research suggests that turmeric may be good for more than just spicing up your diet.

Turmeric (*Curcuma longa*) is a tropical perennial plant that belongs to the ginger (*Zingiberaceae*) family. Turmeric is native to Asia and thrives in clay-like soil in warm, wet climates. Turmeric was first cultivated over 5,000 years ago in what is present-day Pakistan, but it wasn't introduced to the Western world until the thirteenth century. Today, 90 percent of all turmeric is produced in India—not surprising, since India is the world's largest exporter and consumer of the spice.

Commercial turmeric is produced from the plant's rhizome, a horizontal underground stem with knobby fingerlike branches. The rhizome is cleaned, boiled, dried and ground into powder. Turmeric powder has been used for thousands of years as a seasoning, as a preservative, as a dye and as a medicine.

# An Ancient Cure for Modern Times

Turmeric is an important herb in Ayurveda, an ancient Indian healing tradition that is one of the oldest medical systems in the world. According to Ayurvedic tradition, turmeric has many uses: relieving pain, regulating menstruation, aiding digestion, supporting liver health and more.

Turmeric also plays a role in traditional Chinese medicine (TCM), where it is used to regulate the *qi*, or life force. Chinese healers use turmeric to provide topical pain relief and to support blood flow, bile production and digestive health. TCM practitioners also consider turmeric a powerful anti-inflammatory.

Curcumin, the main active constituent of turmeric, is a powerful antioxidant, and many of turmeric's health benefits are linked to antioxidant activity; in fact, researchers from the Indian Agricultural Research Institute evaluated the antioxidant activity of 36 Asian vegetables and found turmeric to be the most potent. But modern research has also found turmeric to have anti-inflammatory, antispasmodic and antibacterial properties. Turmeric may even heal wounds and fight tumors.

## Turmeric and Cancer

In 1992, researchers from the Cancer Research Institute in Bombay, India, studied the effects of curcumin on cancer in mice. Their findings, published in the *Journal of the American College of Nutrition*, showed that curcumin could inhibit cancer initiation, promotion and progression.

In the same year, researchers from India's National Institute of Nutrition examined the effects of curcumin on mutagens in smokers.

(Mutagens, molecules that alter genetic information, are frequently carcinogenic.) After giving 16 chronic smokers 1.5 grams of turmeric daily for 30 days, the researchers reported a reduction in the smokers' urinary mutagen excretions.

Research on turmeric and cancer is not limited to India. In 2005, researchers at the United Kingdom's University of Leicester investigated the potential use of curcumin for humans with colon cancer. For seven days, patients with colorectal cancer received a capsule containing curcumin (some received 450 milligrams, some 1.8 grams and others 3.6 grams). The researchers reported that a 3.6-gram dose of curcumin reduced levels of M(1)G (a biomarker for cancer) in colorectal tissue.

## Turmeric and Digestive Health

In 2001, faculty from the department of pharmacology at Mahidol University in Bangkok, Thailand, used turmeric to treat 25 patients with peptic ulcers. The researchers gave each patient five 600 milligram doses of turmeric per day: before each meal, at 4 PM, and at bedtime. After four weeks, ulcers had healed in 12 patients (48 percent); after eight weeks, ulcers had healed in 18 patients (72 percent); and after 12 weeks, ulcers had healed in 19 patients (76 percent)—a significant improvement over the typical 40 percent rate of spontaneous healing for untreated ulcers.

In 2003, after finding that curcumin reduced symptoms and inflammatory markers in mice with inflamed colons, researchers at the Indian Institute of Chemical Biology suggested curcumin as a treatment for irritable bowel disease.

In 2004, the *Journal of Complementary and Alternative Medicine* published the results of a randomized pilot study of the effects of turmeric extract on irritable bowel syndrome (IBS) symptoms. In this study, researchers gave 207 subjects with IBS one or two tablets of turmeric daily for eight weeks. After treatment, symptoms improved in roughly two-thirds of the subjects.

## Turmeric, Blood Sugar and Diabetes

Diabetes is becoming an epidemic in the United States—the National Institute of Diabetes and Digestive and Kidney Diseases reports that 23.6 million Americans (nearly 8 percent of the population) had diabetes in 2007. Animal studies suggest that turmeric may be helpful for diabetes and related complications, although clinical studies have yet to confirm the findings.

The September 2008 issue of *Molecular Nutrition & Food Research* reported a study on the effects of curcumin on blood glucose and insulin in mice. Korean researchers fed diabetic and non-diabetic mice curcumin for six weeks (mice in the control group received no curcumin). Curcumin significantly lowered blood glucose levels in the diabetic mice, but not in the non-diabetic mice. These findings suggest that curcumin may play a role in glucose control for type 2 diabetes.

In 2007, researchers at Wayne State University in Michigan found that curcumin may help prevent diabetic retinopathy, a common complication in diabetics and a leading cause of blindness in the United States. In a placebo-controlled study, the researchers fed diabetic rats curcumin for six weeks and then examined the rat's retinas for signs of inflammation and oxidative stress. They found that curcumin protected the rats' eyes by preventing diabetes from reducing the antioxidant capacity of the retinas.

Curcumin may also protect against other complications associated with diabetes. In 1995, Indian researchers reported that curcumin improved metabolic health in diabetic rats. In 1998, the same researchers found that eight weeks of curcumin supplementation improved symptoms of diabetes-related kidney damage in rats.

## Turmeric and Cardiovascular Health

In 1992, researchers at the Amala Cancer Research Centre in India conducted a small clinical trial to evaluate the effects of curcumin on cholesterol levels and lipid peroxides (oxidized fatty acids). Ten volunteers received 500 milligrams of curcumin per day for seven days. At the end of the study, the volunteers showed decreased levels of lipid peroxides and cholesterol, and increased levels of HDL ("good") cholesterol. Based on these findings, the researchers recommended further research on the potential use of curcumin to prevent arterial disease.

In 2005, Hossam Arafa, a researcher at Al-Azhar University in Cairo, Egypt, studied the effects of curcumin on blood lipid levels in rats. Arafa fed rats a high-cholesterol diet for seven days, raising their blood lipid and LDL ("bad") cholesterol levels while lowering their HDL cholesterol levels. Arafa then introduced curcumin to the rats' diets, which reversed many of the damaging effects of the high-cholesterol diet, lowering blood lipid and LDL levels while raising HDL levels. Arafa concluded that curcumin has obvious cholesterol-lowering effects unrelated to its antioxidant activity.

## Turmeric and the Mind

Alzheimer's disease is a degenerative brain disease that affects memory and other cognitive functions. Though it is associated with age, Alzheimer's disease is not a normal part of aging. Researchers have identified several risk factors for Alzheimer's disease, including

## A SPICE BY ANY OTHER NAME

The authors of *Turmeric: The Genus Curcuma* report that turmeric has 55 names in Sanskrit, each describing the spice's medicinal and religious uses. A few of these names, along with their meanings, are listed below:

*Ranjani*: that which gives color

*Mangal prada*: auspicious, lucky

*Krimighni*: killing worms (refers to turmeric's antimicrobial action)

*Hemaragi*: being the color of gold

*Varna-datri*: that which gives color (refers to turmeric's ability to enhance the complexion)

*Pavitra*: holy

*Hridayavilasani*: delighting the heart

genetics, environmental toxins, oxidation and inflammation.

Because of its antioxidant and anti-inflammatory properties, some researchers hypothesize that turmeric may reduce the risk of Alzheimer's disease. This hypothesis is supported by the low rates of Alzheimer's disease in India, where turmeric is a common spice and Alzheimer's disease affects as little as one percent of the elderly populations in some villages.

Research on animals explains how turmeric protects against Alzheimer's disease. A team of researchers at the University of California, Los Angeles, conducted one such study in 2001, testing the effects of curcumin on inflammation, oxidation and plaque buildup in mice with symptoms of Alzheimer's. Curcumin decreased all three, leading the researchers to conclude that curcumin shows promise as a preventive treatment for Alzheimer's disease.

## Turmeric and Arthritis

Arthritis, or joint inflammation, causes pain and limits movement. There are more than 100 types of arthritis, all of which involve degeneration of the cartilage that normally protects joints. Often, arthritis is caused by injury, infection or wear and tear. Sometimes, as in cases of rheumatoid arthritis, it is caused by autoimmune responses in which the body attacks its own cells.

Because of its anti-inflammatory properties, some researchers have considered turmeric as a potential treatment for arthritis. In 2006, researchers at the Center for Phytomedicine Research at the University of Arizona used turmeric to treat rats with symptoms of rheumatoid arthritis. Some of the rats received treatment before the onset of symptoms, and some of the rats after. The researchers found that an extract containing primarily curcuminoids (including curcumin) reduced joint swelling, but only when treatment was given before the onset of symptoms. The researchers concluded that curcuminoids are responsible for turmeric's antiarthritic action.

# Where to Get Your Turmeric

Turmeric is available in capsules, liquid extracts and tinctures—even in teas, thanks to the spice's growing popularity. Many turmeric supplements contain bromelain, an enzyme derived from pineapple that improves the absorption and anti-inflammatory action of curcumin. For those using supplements, alternative health guru Dr. Andrew Weil recommends 400 to 600 milligrams of turmeric extract three times a day. Or, you can skip the pills and bottles and simply enjoy more curries and Indian food. Whichever route you take, your body is sure to thank you.

# The Bottom Line

Turmeric is a delicious and widely available spice with numerous health benefits. Whether you take it as a supplement or use it to spice up your diet, turmeric provides a healthy dose of antioxidants that may help prevent or provide relief for chronic conditions such as Alzheimer's disease, arthritis, cardiovascular disease and more. There's a reason cultures around the world have used turmeric for thousands of years—so go ahead and have another dish of curry.

## TURMERIC FAST FACTS

**Uses and Benefits:** Turmeric may reduce inflammation and cholesterol; relieve symptoms of inflammatory bowel disease (IBD), rheumatoid arthritis and cystic fibrosis; prevent cancer and Alzheimer's disease; and support liver and cardiovascular function.

**Sources:** Turmeric is a common spice and is featured prominently in curries and many Middle Eastern cuisines. Turmeric supplements are available as capsules, liquids, tinctures and teas.

**Special Considerations:** Look for supplements with bromelain, which may increase absorption and improve the anti-inflammatory action of curcumin.

Turmeric is generally considered safe and nontoxic. Some people may experience allergic reactions to turmeric, including skin irritation and anaphylaxis, though such reactions are rare.

# 17

# Vitamin B

The B vitamin family comprises eight water-soluble nutrients that are essential for functions and processes throughout the body. Most of us probably take the B vitamins for granted, but if we understood how important they are to our well-being, we would be sure to get adequate daily amounts, both from our diet and from nutritional supplements.

## Eight Vitamins for a Thousand Functions

Like vitamin C and other water-soluble vitamins, B vitamins are absorbed directly into the bloodstream. Because the body excretes excess water-soluble vitamins through the urine, we must consume B vitamins regularly. (Fat-soluble vitamins such as vitamins A and D are stored in fat reserves and released into the bloodstream as needed.)

Every B vitamin is necessary for metabolizing proteins, fats and carbohydrates. B vitamins perform thousands of other functions throughout the body, including the creation of metabolic coenzymes, which help enzymes facilitate critical reactions. Some B vitamins facilitate energy-releasing reactions, while some help build new cells that deliver nutrients to others.

Among their many benefits, B vitamins can help alleviate menstrual and PMS symptoms, prevent mild depression, regulate heart function, lower blood levels of homocysteine, prevent nervous system dysfunction and prevent (or lessen) the effects of diabetes. Folic-acid supplementation lowers the incidence of birth defects, and B-complex vitamins in general have been shown to reduce health risks in children whose mothers take them while pregnant and lactating. In various studies, B vitamins have been shown to reduce babies' susceptibility to diabetes, obesity, spina bifida and possibly even cancer.

B vitamins are usually sold individually or as B-complex supplements, which typically contain all eight B vitamins. To clarify the role and function of each B-vitamin family, let's review the actions and benefits of each nutrient.

---

### The B-vitamin family

- B1—Thiamine
- B2—Riboflavin
- B3—Niacin
- B5—Pantothenic Acid
- B6—Pyridoxine
- B7—Biotin
- B9—Folic Acid
- B12—Cyanocobalamin

---

## Vitamin B1—Thiamine

To better understand what thiamine does in the body, consider the word that describes thiamine deficiency: *beriberi*. This Sinhalese word means, "I can't, I can't." And people suffering from beriberi can't do a lot. They are weak, fatigued and without appetite. They may have burning feet, cramps and mental confusion. But beriberi patients, even at the brink of death, suffering from severe fluid retention and completely incapacitated, can be on their feet and almost completely recovered within a couple hours after receiving a thiamine injection. Thiamine is essential for energy production.

## Thiamine and Brain Function

Thiamine's role in energy production has ramifications for the brain as well. Dramatically reduced thiamine intake severely limits the brain's ability to use glucose. Without glucose, brain function becomes slow and impaired.

Thiamine is also used to synthesize critical neurotransmitters such as acetylcholine, which is involved in memory, mood and mental performance. In an article published in the journal *Psychopharmacology*, researchers investigated the effects of long-term supplementation with nine vitamins, including thiamine. After 12 months, the researchers found that thiamine improved attention in female subjects. (Interestingly, the same effect did not occur in male subjects, although the researchers could not explain this difference.)

In another study, published in the *Journal of Gerontology*, researchers reported that thiamine supplementation decreased fatigue and increased energy, appetite and general well-being in elderly women with mild thiamine deficiencies.

# Vitamin B2—Riboflavin

Riboflavin participates in the production of adenosine triphosphate (ATP), the body's basic energy currency. The body uses ATP any time energy is needed—to move muscles, digest food, breathe, make protein, etc. If riboflavin is in short supply, our energy reserves become depleted and we become lethargic.

Riboflavin also helps the body produce glutathione, a potent anti-oxidant. Research suggests that riboflavin deficiencies may be associated with the development of cataracts, possibly because glutathione protects the eyes against cellular damage caused by sunlight and other factors.

Riboflavin supplementation may also help prevent and treat migraine headaches. Researchers from the University of Liège, in Belgium, found that riboflavin was more effective than the placebo at reducing the frequency and duration of migraine headaches. More recently, the same researchers published the results of a study indicating that riboflavin provided benefits to migraine patients similar to the benefits provided by beta-blockers (a class of medication). The researchers also observed that riboflavin and beta blockers acted through different mechanisms and might therefore have complementary functions.

# Vitamin B3—Niacin

Niacin plays many roles in the body, including helping enzymes convert food into energy. These same enzymes also help the body manufacture hormones and metabolize fat and cholesterol. Niacin contributes to the process of DNA repair and the stability of genomes and helps boost overall immune system health.

## Niacin: Heart Helper

Research shows that niacin—in the form of nicotinic acid—helps to reduce total cholesterol levels and raise HDL ("good") cholesterol levels. In the Coronary Drug Project, more than 8,000 male subjects took either three grams of nicotinic acid or a placebo every day for six years. The researchers conducting the study found that nicotinic acid significantly decreased total cholesterol and triglyceride levels and reduced the risk of heart attack and stroke.

One note of caution: Consult with your physician before using supplemental niacin to lower total cholesterol and raise HDL cholesterol levels—high doses of niacin have been linked to liver damage.

# Vitamin B5—Pantothenic Acid

Pantothenic acid is very common—its name comes from the Greek root *pantos*, which means "everywhere." Pantothenic acid is involved in over a hundred critical body processes, including energy production and the manufacture of steroids, hormones, neurotransmitters and hemoglobin.

## Pantothenic Acid and Coenzyme A

Pantothenic acid is an essential component of coenzyme A, a catalyst for many chemical reactions. Coenzyme A plays a broad role in producing energy and distributing glucose, fatty acids and proteins throughout the body. Our bodies also use coenzyme A to detoxify tissues.

## Other Uses of Pantothenic Acid

Preliminary research indicates that calcium D-pantothenate (a form of pantothenic acid) may enhance wound healing. Additionally, pantethine, a derivative of pantothenic acid, may reduce cholesterol and triglyceride levels.

# Vitamin B6—Pyridoxine

There are three forms of vitamin B6: pyridoxine, pyridoxal and pyridoxamine. All three are present in most body tissues, with the highest concentration being in the liver. Of the three, pyridoxine is the most resistant to food processing and storage conditions and is thus the most prevalent form in most diets.

Vitamin B6 is involved in dozens of vital physiological processes. It plays a primary role in protein metabolism, helps form hemoglobin, aids in the absorption of amino acids from the intestine and helps metabolize fats and carbohydrates.

Several studies have linked vitamin B6 deficiency with heart disease. For example, researchers from the Harvard School of Public Health found that women with higher intakes of vitamin B6 had less risk of coronary heart disease. The cardio-protective properties of vitamin B6 may be related to the vitamin's role in regulating blood levels of homocysteine, a substance associated with cardiovascular disease.

Vitamin B6 deficiency has been associated with Alzheimer's disease. Additionally, researchers at Tufts University in Boston have reported a positive association between vitamin B6 status and memory in older men.

Research shows that vitamin B6 plays a definitive role in regulating the hormones estrogen, progesterone, testosterone and glucocorticoid (a stress hormone). This may explain why vitamin B6 provides relief for women with morning sickness.

Vitamin B6 deficiency may increase the risk of cancer in smokers and has been linked to rheumatoid arthritis, kidney stones and carpal tunnel syndrome. Studies also show that vitamin B6 may help alleviate asthma symptoms.

# Vitamin B7—Biotin

Biotin acts as a coenzyme that helps transport carbon dioxide between compounds. Biotin also plays a role in protein synthesis, the formation of long-chain fatty acids and the Krebs cycle, the basic biological process that releases energy from food.

Most people aren't deficient in biotin; however, deficiency may occur in people who suffer from absorption problems such as Crohn's disease. Additionally, some infants suffer from a genetic disorder that interferes with their ability to absorb biotin.

Biotin is best known for its role in strengthening fingernails and hair by helping the body utilize fatty acids to create keratin, the protein that comprises nails and hair.

Biotin supplementation also shows promise for diabetics. Several studies show that biotin can enhance the performance of insulin. In one small study, researchers found that a 16,000 mcg daily dose of biotin decreased blood glucose levels in people with type 1 diabetes after one week. In another study, researchers found that a 9,000 mcg daily dose of biotin decreased fasting blood glucose levels by approximately 50 percent in people with type 2 diabetics after one month of treatment.

# Vitamin B9—Folic Acid (Folate)

The terms folate and folic acid are used interchangeably when referring to vitamin B9. Folic acid is the more stable of the two forms and is often found in supplements and fortified foods. Folate occurs naturally in food sources such as spinach and other green leafy vegetables. Like other B vitamins, folic acid is necessary for a variety of functions and body processes, from cellular maintenance to the prevention of birth defects in developing fetuses.

## Folic Acid and DNA and RNA Synthesis

Folic acid is essential for the synthesis of DNA, the genetic blueprint that allows cells to properly develop and divide. Doctors recommend that pregnant women take folic acid supplements, a practice that has significantly reduced the incidence of certain birth defects. Researchers at the University of California, Berkeley, have found that even mild folic acid deficiency can greatly increase the incidence of damaged DNA. Other studies have linked folic acid deficiencies to the development of dysplasia (abnormal cell development often linked to cancer) in the colon, the lungs and the cervix.

## Folic Acid and Homocysteine

Recent studies indicate that folic acid, taken alone or with other B vitamins, can effectively lower homocysteine levels. Homocysteine is associated with atherosclerosis and myocardial infarction, as well inflammation associated with rheumatoid arthritis. In addition, excess homocysteine can significantly add to the amount of stress a person experiences. B vitamin supplements can help bring homocysteine levels down and may reduce stress.

## How Much Folic Acid Do We Need?

Research shows that most of us aren't getting enough folic acid in our diets. Most people consume about 200 micrograms of folic acid each day. This is only half of the daily recommendation, and many experts believe the daily recommendation is inadequate. Good food sources of folic acid include green leafy vegetables, lentils, pinto, navy, lima and kidney beans, tuna, oranges, strawberries, wheat germ, asparagus, bananas, and cantaloupe. Eat these foods as fresh as possible, because heat and long storage times can destroy folic acid content.

# Vitamin B12—Cyanocobalamin

Vitamin B12 is composed of several compounds that are given the generic name cobalamins because all of them contain cobalt. Vitamin B12 cannot be synthesized by plants and is found primarily in meat and meat products. This is why vegetarians, and especially vegans, can have vitamin B12 deficiencies.

Vitamin B12 is necessary for the proper function of every cell in your body. It is also necessary for DNA and RNA synthesis, and the body needs additional vitamin B12 in areas where cells reproduce frequently, such as the blood and intestines. Without adequate vitamin B12, cells cannot divide and multiply. This can lead to anemia. In the intestines, it can mean a reduction in the absorption of nutrients, potentially causing other nutrient deficiencies. Vitamin B12 is useful in several other ways, including:

In some parts of the body, a shortage of vitamin B12 can interfere with cell growth, and the resulting cell abnormalities can eventually lead to cancer. Several studies have found an inverse relation between vitamin B12 status and breast cancer risk, especially in postmenopausal women.

B12 helps maintain myelin, the fatty sheath that surrounds and protects nerve fibers and promotes their normal growth. A B12 deficiency can cause myelin to break down, resulting in nerve damage, which can then contribute to serious nervous system problems. Various problems have been linked to vitamin B12 deficiency, including memory loss, confusion, delusion, fatigue, loss of balance, numbness and tingling in the hands, ringing in the ears and decreased reflexes. B12 deficiency has also been linked to multiple sclerosis–like symptoms and dementia.

Research indicates that vitamin B12 deficiency raises the levels of homocysteine, which has been suggested as a cause of heart disease, heart attack, and stroke. Vitamin B12 supplements can reduce homocysteine levels, which may reduce chronic stress.

# The Bottom Line

The B vitamins are vital for good health. A deficiency of any of them can create a domino effect resulting in various health problems. B vitamins are crucial to proper body functioning, from creating and maintaining energy production to assisting enzymes in their many functions and assisting in the creation of red blood cells. B-vitamin deficiencies are linked to a host of ailments, including heart disease, dementia and cancer. A well-rounded diet can provide adequate amounts of B vitamins, but ample research suggests that many people do not get enough B vitamins; thus, B-complex supplements may help treat and prevent a wide variety of diseases and promote overall health.

## VITAMINS FAST FACTS

**Uses and Benefits:** The benefits of B vitamins are wide-ranging, from prevention of heart disease and relief from depression and stress to cancer prevention and reduced symptoms of PMS. Additionally, all B vitamins are involved in myriad body processes that are essential for good health.

**Sources:** B-complex supplements or daily multivitamin/mineral supplements. Specific B vitamins are also sold individually.

**Special Considerations:** Because most B vitamins work synergistically, it's best to take either a B-complex supplement or a multivitamin/mineral supplement with the full complement of B vitamins. Only take individual B-vitamin supplements if you know you're deficient or if you have a specific disorder that would require therapeutic doses. Always consult with a qualified health care provider before beginning any such therapy.

# 18

# Vitamin C

Vitamin C is perhaps the most widely known and most popular of all nutrients. Also called ascorbic acid, vitamin C is a water-soluble vitamin and a powerful antioxidant. Vitamin C is involved in hundreds of body processes, including collagen production, immune system regulation, blood vessel maintenance, cell repair and hormone production.

Most animals synthesize vitamin C from glucose and other sugars, but humans do not have this ability. All human vitamin C requirements must be met through diet or supplementation. Since vitamin C is water soluble, the body stores only small amounts and excretes excess quantities in the urine. Because of this, everyone should ensure an adequate daily intake of foods rich in vitamin C. Vitamin C is a highly unstable compound that rapidly deteriorates in storage and food preparation, so fresh fruits and vegetables are the best sources.

Vitamin C is well known today, but its discovery was surprisingly recent. The Hungarian biochemist Albert Szent-Györgi first isolated vitamin C in 1928 and won the Nobel Prize in 1938 for his discovery.

But while vitamin C itself was unknown before 1938, a *lack* of vitamin C—manifest as the disease scurvy—has plagued humankind for millennia. The first known record of scurvy dates from the sixteenth century BCE and describes classic symptoms such as gum inflammation, tooth decay, lack of energy and bleeding problems. It wasn't until the seventeenth century CE—over 3,000 years later—that the British surgeon James Lind discovered that lemons and limes could prevent and cure the deadly disease. Scurvy was common among sailors, and after Lind's discovery, British ships began to carry limes for the sailors to eat, earning British sailors the nickname "limeys." While scurvy is rare in Western industrialized society today, it is still a problem in developing areas of the world.

# Functions of Vitamin C

## *Antioxidant*

Because of its powerful antioxidant properties, vitamin C plays an important role in neutralizing free radicals throughout the body. In addition, vitamin C protects the fat-soluble antioxidants vitamins A and E from excessive oxidation. Scientists theorize that reducing free radical activity in the body can help prevent cell death, protect against cancer and other diseases and slow the aging process.

## *Building Connective Tissue*

The body requires vitamin C to manufacture collagen, a protein that binds the body's cells together. Collagen is the most abundant tissue in the body and is needed to build and maintain skin, tendons, ligaments, muscles and joints. Collagen is also essential in healing wounds, fractures and other injuries.

## Building Strong Teeth and Bones

Vitamin C is needed for calcification, the process of forming bones, and for the manufacture of dentin, a major component in teeth.

## Immune System Function

Vitamin C supports healthy immune system function in several ways. It enhances the function of phagocytes, cells that destroy foreign invaders; it assists in the production of lymphocytes, white blood cells that help fight infection; it helps produce antibodies, substances that protect against bacteria and viruses; and it supports the thymus, an important part of the immune system.

## Metabolism

The body needs vitamin C to properly metabolize fats and some proteins, including tyrosine, which is used to produce adrenaline, dopamine and tryptophan. Vitamin C is also critical for metabolizing folic acid.

## Sources of Vitamin C

The best food sources of vitamin C include citrus fruits (such as lemons, limes, oranges, tangerines, grapefruit, pomelos, clementines and mandarin oranges), citrus juices, cantaloupe and other melons, strawberries, kiwi, mango, papaya, pineapples, red and green bell peppers, tomatoes and tomato juice, Brussels sprouts, cabbage and broccoli. Since vitamin C is such a fragile vitamin, concentrations are highest in fresh, uncooked servings of these foods.

Vitamin C is also available in multivitamins and other dietary supplements. As a single nutrient, vitamin C is available in tablet, capsule, powder, liquid, effervescent and even chewing gum forms. Many people choose to take a daily vitamin C supplement to ensure that their basic dietary needs are met and to help protect against disease.

# Recommended Daily Allowance

The U.S. government recently raised the recommended daily allowance (RDA) of vitamin C for adults from 60 milligrams to 80 milligrams. The following table offers RDAs for specific age and risk groups:

It's important to note that RDAs are based on the amount of vitamin C the body needs to prevent a deficiency that would cause scurvy, rather than the amount needed to prevent disease and promote optimal health. Based on the results of many studies, some scientists now recommend a daily intake of 400 milligrams for healthy adults.

| Life Stage | Age | Male (mg/day) | Female (mg/day) |
|------------|-----|---------------|-----------------|
| Infants | 0-6 months | 40 (AI*) | 40 (AI) |
| Infants | 7-12 months | 50 (AI*) | 50 (AI) |
| Children | 1-3 years | 15 | 15 |
| Children | 4-8 years | 25 | 25 |
| Children | 9-13 years | 45 | 45 |
| Adolescents | 14-18 | 75 | 75 |
| Adults | 19 ≥ | 90 | 90 |
| Smokers | 19 ≥ | 125 | 125 |
| Pregnancy | 18 ≤ | — | 80 |
| Pregnancy | 19 ≥ | — | 85 |
| Breastfeeding | 18≤ | — | 115 |
| Breastfeeding | 19≥ | — | 120 |

*AI: Adequate intake, when exact RDA cannot be determined.
Source: Linus Pauling Institute at Oregon State University

# People with Special Requirements

Some people need more vitamin C because of health, nutrition, and lifestyle concerns. People who are depressed or over-stressed; who drink more than two alcoholic drinks per day; who only eat cooked and processed foods; or who take analgesics, antidepressants, steroids or anticoagulants are well advised to consider a daily vitamin C supplement. Additionally, people who smoke and people older than 65 can benefit from supplemental vitamin C.

# Deficiency

Symptoms of vitamin C deficiency include bleeding gums, easy bruising, joint pain, poor digestion, slow healing of wounds, weight loss and poor resistance to cold, flu, or other infectious diseases. Vitamin C deficiency is rare in the United States today.

# Vitamin C and Disease

Many scientific studies conducted throughout the world over the past 50 years have produced solid evidence correlating adequate vitamin C intake or high levels of vitamin C intake with a reduced risk of many serious diseases and health conditions, including the following:

- Asthma
- Cancer
- Cardiovascular disease
- Cataracts
- Common cold
- Diabetes
- Hypertension
- Parkinson's disease
- Poor immune system function

While the daily doses of vitamin C used in research studies range from 40 milligrams to nine grams (9,000 milligrams), a daily intake from 400 milligrams to 1,000 milligrams should provide maximum benefits in preventing disease and promoting optimal health. If you think you may benefit from additional quantities, please discuss your specific needs with your health care professional.

## Safety

Vitamin C is typically nontoxic in oral doses, but excessive quantities may cause the following symptoms:

- Bloating
- Diarrhea
- Frequent urination
- Flatulence
- Nausea
- Upset stomach

If you are taking supplemental vitamin C and are experiencing any of the above symptoms, reduce your dosage or consult with your health care professional.

## VITAMIN C FAST FACTS

**Uses and Benefits:** Vitamin C plays an important role in the formation of collagen and other structural components of the body. Vitamin C is also a powerful antioxidant that supports healthy metabolism and immune system function. Vitamin C may reduce the risk of many serious diseases, including cancer and cardiovascular disease.

**Sources:** Rich food sources of vitamin C include citrus fruits and juices, melons, strawberries, kiwi, mango, papaya, pineapples, bell peppers, tomatoes and tomato juice, Brussels sprouts, cabbage and broccoli. Vitamin C is a fragile vitamin, so concentrations are highest in fresh, uncooked servings of these foods. Vitamin C is also available in multivitamins and as a single nutrient in tablet, capsule, powder, liquid, effervescent and even chewing gum forms.

**Special Considerations:** Vitamin C is generally considered safe, as the body excretes excess quantities in the urine. However, too much vitamin C may cause bloating, diarrhea, frequent urination, flatulence, nausea or upset stomach.

# 19

# Vitamin D

Vitamin D is a fat-soluble vitamin that the human body uses to maintain normal calcium metabolism and promote bone health. The body can synthesize vitamin D when the skin is exposed to ultraviolet radiation from the sun. Vitamin D can also be obtained from both natural food sources and fortified foods. Vitamin D deficiency can create many health problems, and severe vitamin D deficiency results in a condition known as rickets, a debilitating decalcification of the bones. Rickets was common among American children until the 1940s, when the U.S. government began a widespread program to fortify milk with vitamin D.

Today, important new studies have renewed interest in the role vitamin D plays in maintaining health and preventing disease. Scientific evidence associates vitamin D deficiency with an increased incidence of many diseases—including cancer, cardiovascular disease, osteoporosis, stroke, Parkinson's disease and autoimmune disorders—and suggests that supplemental vitamin D can help prevent these serious health conditions.

New discoveries about vitamin D's role in human health have been so important that *Time* magazine named "The Benefits of Vitamin D" as one of the top ten medical breakthroughs of 2007. Adding his perspective to the excitement, interventional nutrition expert Dr. Greg Plotnikoff doesn't mince words: "Because vitamin D is so cheap and so clearly reduces all-cause mortality, I can say this with great certainty: Vitamin D represents the single most cost-effective medical intervention in the United States."

# Functions

Vitamin D plays a critical role in many physiological processes, including calcium balance, blood pressure regulation, insulin production, cell differentiation and immune system function. Vitamin D's most important functions involve maintaining normal blood levels of calcium, assisting calcium absorption and building bone mass.

# Sources

Vitamin D is available from three basic sources: sunlight, food and supplements. Most people depend on a combination of these sources to meet their needs.

## Sunlight

Exposure to sunlight stimulates the epidermis of the skin to produce vitamin D. In fact, many people meet their entire vitamin D requirement by exposure to the sun. However, people with dark skin and those with limited exposure to sunlight need to be especially careful to ensure that their vitamin D needs are met through diet or supplementation.

## Food Sources

While most vitamins are found abundantly in many of the foods we eat, food sources of vitamin D are quite limited. The best food sources are egg yolks and oily fish such as salmon, mackerel and sardines. Foods with small amounts of vitamin D include oatmeal, parsley, sweet potatoes and dandelion greens.

## Fortified Foods

Because natural food sources of vitamin D are so limited, food manufacturers routinely fortify processed foods with vitamin D. The U.S. government initiated fortification in response to the high incidence of rickets among children in the first half of the twentieth century. In fact, in the 1920s, 75 percent of children in New York Public Schools had some form of rickets. In the 1940s, U.S. dairies began fortifying milk with vitamin D, which led to drastic reductions in the incidence of rickets in the U.S. population.

Today, the foods most commonly fortified with vitamin D include milk, orange juice, yogurt and breakfast cereals. Eight ounces of milk or fortified orange juice contain 100 IU of vitamin D, and a one-cup serving of fortified breakfast cereal contains 40 to 50 IU. Not all breakfast cereals or brands of orange juice are fortified with vitamin D, so it's important to read the labels to determine exact vitamin D content.

## Dietary Supplements

Vitamin D is also available in supplement form, either as part of multivitamin formulas or as an individual supplement. Taking a vitamin D supplement is the easiest and most effective way to ensure an adequate intake of vitamin D.

# Recommended Daily Intake

## *Adults*

Nutritionists once based recommendations for daily vitamin D intake solely on the amount needed to prevent rickets. But because scientists now recognize vitamin D's role in so many critical physiological functions, experts now recommend 200 IU for adults under 50, 400 IU for adults ages 51 to 70, and 600 IU for adults over 70.

## *Infants and Children*

In 2008, the American Academy of Pediatrics (AAP) revised its recommended daily intake of vitamin D for infants and children to 400 IU. Additionally, the AAP recommends vitamin D supplements for breast-fed and partially breast-fed infants as well as non-breast-fed infants and children who drink less than one liter of vitamin-D–fortified milk or formula per day.

# Deficiency

## *Symptoms of Deficiency*

Symptoms of vitamin D deficiency include muscle pain, muscle twitching, visual problems, bone pain, anemia, diarrhea, joint pain, insomnia, nervousness and a burning sensation in the mouth. If you have any of these symptoms and suspect a deficiency, consult with your physician for proper diagnosis and treatment.

## *Who's at Risk?*

Several population groups in the United States are at particular risk for vitamin D deficiency. These groups fall broadly into several categories, including people with limited sun exposure, the elderly, people with certain health conditions, exclusively breast-fed infants and people taking certain medications.

## Those with limited sun exposure

Sunlight exposure alone provides many with sufficient quantities of vitamin D, but people with dark skin and limited exposure to the sun should be especially careful to ensure adequate vitamin D intake from diet and supplements. People who live in northern latitudes and those who routinely protect themselves from the sun with sunscreen and clothing are especially prone to vitamin D deficiency.

## The elderly

As we age, our ability to synthesize vitamin D from sunlight decreases, resulting in lower vitamin D levels. Additionally, the elderly are more likely to spend time indoors and out of the sun. For older adults, the benefits of supplemental vitamin D in preventing disease and prolonging life are especially important.

## Those with health conditions

Several health conditions can affect the absorption and metabolism of vitamin D. People with these conditions should consult with their physician to determine appropriate supplementation strategies. These conditions include obesity, fat malabsorption syndromes (such as cystic fibrosis and cholestatic liver disease), inflammatory bowel disease and Crohn's disease.

## Exclusively breast-fed infants

Human milk contains only 25 IU of vitamin D per liter, so exclusively breast-fed infants need supplemental vitamin D to reach the recommended daily intake of 400 IU.

## *Those taking medications*

Certain medications can interfere with vitamin D absorption. These medications include barbiturates, corticosteroids, antacids and statins (cholesterol-lowering drugs). People taking these medications should consider vitamin D supplementation to ensure sufficient intake.

# Overall Mortality

An important study published in the *Archives of Internal Medicine* in 2008 reveals that inadequate vitamin D intake significantly increases overall mortality. In the study, researchers at Johns Hopkins University followed a group of 13,000 initially healthy men and women for more than eight years. During this period, 1,806 people died, including 400 who were deficient in vitamin D. Lead author Dr. Michal Melamed summarized the study's results: "Those who had the lowest levels of vitamin D had a 26 percent higher risk of death from all causes compared to those with the highest vitamin D levels."

# Disease Prevention

Scientists have long recognized the importance of vitamin D in human health, but recent studies have forced the medical world to reevaluate the role vitamin D plays in preventing disease. Dr. Michael F. Holick, director of the Vitamin D, Skin and Bone Research Laboratory at Boston University Medical Center, said, "We know that being vitamin D sufficient reduces the risk of having your first heart attack by more than 50 percent, reduces the risk of having peripheral vascular disease by as much as 80 percent, and decreases the risk of prostate, colon, breast and a whole host of other cancers by as much as 50 to 70 percent."

## Osteoporosis

Vitamin D deficiency can contribute to the development of osteoporosis. A 2006 multinational study of 2,600 postmenopausal women with osteoporosis found that 64 percent of the participants had insufficient blood levels of vitamin D. Additionally, in a 2003 study published in the *American Journal of Clinical Nutrition*, researchers followed 72,000 women for 18 years and found that the women who consumed at least 600 IU per day of vitamin D had a 37 percent lower risk of osteoporosis-related hip fracture than women who consumed less than 140 IU per day. Other clinical trials offer additional evidence that vitamin D supplementation reduces bone density loss and osteoporotic fractures in adults who are deficient.

Current evidence suggests that a minimum daily intake of 600 IU of vitamin D can reduce the incidence of bone decalcification and fractures among the elderly. Those who take supplemental vitamin D to promote bone health and avoid fractures should also ensure an adequate dietary intake of calcium (1,000 to 1,200 milligrams per day).

## Cancer

Scientists have found positive links between vitamin D deficiency and several types of cancer, including breast cancer, prostate cancer and colon cancer. A 2007 study of 1,179 postmenopausal women revealed that participants who took supplements containing 1,100 IU of vitamin D and 1,400 mg of calcium over a period of four years had an overall cancer rate that was 60 percent lower than participants who took only placebos. Study leader Joan Lappe of Creighton University summarized the results: "This clinical trial strongly supports the observational studies that have associated sunlight and vitamin D levels with a lower risk of cancer."

## Cardiovascular Disease

Several recent studies offer strong evidence that low vitamin D levels are correlated with the incidence of cardiovascular disease. In a 2008 study published in the *Archives of Internal Medicine,* researchers compared 454 men (aged 40 to 75) who had a history of heart disease with 900 men who had no history of heart disease. Researchers found that participants with deficient vitamin D levels had a higher risk of heart attack than those with higher vitamin D levels. In another study—one of the most important to date—researchers followed 1,739 members of the Framingham Offspring Study for five years and found that the incidence of cardiovascular disease—including heart attacks, heart failure, and strokes—was from 53 to 80 percent higher in people with low blood levels of vitamin D.

## Stroke

According to the American Heart Association, over half a million Americans have a stroke each year. The most common risk factors for stroke include smoking, high blood pressure, lack of exercise and heart disease. But the results of a study published in 2008 in the journal *Stroke* suggest that the incidence of stroke is higher among people with low vitamin D levels, indicating a correlation between low vitamin D levels and stroke. In another study, a Cambridge University neurologist compared blood vitamin D levels of 34 stroke patients with those of 96 healthy volunteers. Results show that the stroke patients' blood vitamin D levels were a third lower than those of the healthy volunteers.

## Parkinson's Disease

Parkinson's disease is a serious, debilitating health condition that causes stiffness, tremors, and slowness of movement due to inadequate levels of dopamine in the brain. In a 2008 study, researchers at the Emory University School of Medicine found that low vitamin D levels may be associated with Parkinson's disease. In the study, researchers found that 55 percent of Parkinson's patients had insufficient vitamin D levels, compared with 36 percent in a group of healthy elderly participants. Lead researcher Marian Evatt, MD, summarized the results: "We found that vitamin D insufficiency may have a unique association with Parkinson's, which is intriguing and warrants further investigation."

## Autoimmune Diseases

Autoimmune diseases (such as rheumatoid arthritis, multiple sclerosis, and type 1 diabetes) occur when the body launches an immune attack against its own tissues. Researchers have found that one type of immune cell, T cells, are responsible for mediating immune response, and that vitamin D is an important modulator of immune response, thus potentially diminishing the severity of autoimmune diseases. Animal studies confirm that vitamin D therapy can be beneficial in cases of rheumatoid arthritis, type 1 diabetes and multiple sclerosis.

# Safety

According to the American Dietetic Association, the daily tolerable upper intake level of vitamin D for children and adults is 2,000 IU. To prevent vitamin D toxicity and any long-term damage it may cause, do not exceed the 2,000 IU daily limit. Additionally, people who eat large quantities of fish or drink large amounts of fortified milk should use caution when taking supplemental vitamin D.

Long-term, excessive vitamin D intake can lead to serious health conditions, including bone loss; calcification of the heart, lungs, and kidneys; and deafness due to calcification of the tympanic membrane of the ear.

Possible symptoms of vitamin D toxicity include nausea, excessive thirst, appetite loss, dizziness and headaches. If you think you may be suffering from vitamin D toxicity, please see your physician. In addition, individuals with gout, rheumatoid arthritis and hyperthyroidism should consult with their physician before taking more than 400 IU of vitamin D per day.

## Drug Interactions

To avoid any possible drug interactions, please talk with your physician before taking a vitamin D supplement with any of the following medications: orlistat (Xenical), cholestyramine (Questran), ketoconazole and colestipol (Colestid).

# The Bottom Line

Most of us aren't getting enough sunshine, and that means not enough vitamin D. Our health may be suffering as a result. Vitamin D is essential to many bodily functions and may even prevent serious chronic illnesses. Make sure you're getting enough vitamin D by enjoying the sunshine and by taking a daily vitamin D supplement.

## VITAMIN D FAST FACTS

**Uses and Benefits:** Vitamin D is essential for normal calcium metabolism and acts as a potent immune system modulator. Vitamin D plays a role in insulin secretion under some circumstances and may reduce the risk of high blood pressure. Vitamin D may also help prevent osteoporosis, some cancers and some autoimmune diseases.

**Sources:** The primary source of vitamin D is the sun's ultraviolet rays, which stimulate vitamin D–production in the skin. Food sources of vitamin D are limited and include eggs and fatty fish. Milk is often fortified with vitamin D, as is some orange juice and some cereals. Vitamin D supplements are available at your local health food store.

**Special Considerations:** Vitamin D is fat soluble and excess amounts are stored in the body; too much vitamin D can lead to toxicity (hypervitaminosis D), which may cause abnormally high calcium levels (hypercalcemia). If left untreated, hypercalcemia may cause bone loss, kidney stones, and calcification of the heart, kidneys and other organs.

# 20

# Vitamin K

Vitamin K is a fat-soluble vitamin that the body uses for blood clotting and bone formation. The "K" in vitamin K comes from the German word *koagulation*, because the vitamin is essential for the synthesis of proteins that are required for blood coagulation. There are three different forms of vitamin K: vitamin K1 (phylloquinone), which is found in plant foods containing chlorophyll; vitamin K2 (menaquinone), which is found in animal foods and is also synthesized by bacteria in the human gut; and vitamin K3 (menadione), a synthetic form that is not found in nature. Vitamins K1 and K2 both have roles as dietary supplements in recommended amounts, but vitamin K3 is not used as a dietary supplement.

## Sources

Good food sources of vitamin K include dark leafy greens, such as spinach, broccoli and kale, and vegetable oils, such as canola oil, soybean oil, olive oil and cottonseed oil. Additionally, some fruits, nuts and vegetables contain small amounts. One cup of dark leafy greens provides about 120 micrograms of vitamin K, the recommended daily intake for adult men. Most multivitamins contain the recommended daily amount of vitamin K, and further supplementation is typically not needed. However, vitamin K1 (phylloquinone) and K2 (menaquinone) supplements are available at health food stores and are useful in cases of specific health conditions.

# Recommended Daily Intake

The American Dietetic Association recommends a daily vitamin K intake of 75 micrograms for teenagers aged 14 to 18, 90 micrograms for women, and 120 micrograms for men. Most people's vitamin K needs are easily met through diet alone. Individuals taking anticoagulants (blood-thinning drugs) should be careful to eat vitamin K–rich foods in moderation, as too much vitamin K can interfere with the action of their medication.

# Deficiency

Although vitamin K deficiency is rare in the United States, a true deficiency interferes with blood clotting. Symptoms of deficiency include various types of excessive bleeding, such as blood in the urine, nosebleeds, bleeding gums, heavy menstrual bleeding, or tarry, (black stools). If you suspect you may be suffering from a vitamin K deficiency, please contact your physician for proper diagnosis and treatment.

## *Infant Hemorrhagic Disease*

In 1961, the American Academy of Pediatrics recommended that all newborn babies receive an injection of vitamin K to prevent hemorrhagic disease, a condition that interferes with blood coagulation. Since infants are born with a sterile intestinal tract, and a major source of vitamin K is gut bacteria, it takes some time until infants' gut bacteria can colonize and produce adequate levels of vitamin K. The practice of vitamin K supplementation at birth has dramatically reduced the incidence of hemorrhagic disease among infants in the United States.

# Vitamin K and Coagulation

Scientists refer to the process of blood clotting as the coagulation cascade, a series of interdependent events that stop bleeding though the formation of clots. The body utilizes seven different clotting factors, or proteins, in the coagulation cascade, and vitamin K is required to activate these seven factors. If the body lacks adequate amounts of vitamin K to activate the seven clotting factors, blood clots cannot form, leading to life-threatening bleeding disorders.

# Vitamin K and Cardiovascular Disease

Preliminary research suggests that inadequate vitamin K intake may be correlated with an increased incidence of aortic calcification, leading to the development of arteriosclerosis. In a population-based study published in 1995 in the journal *Atherosclerosis*, researchers followed 256 postmenopausal women and found an inverse correlation between long-term intake of vitamin K and arterosclerotic aorta calcification; in other words, the women with lower vitamin-K levels had more aortic calcification than those with higher levels.

In a 2004 study, Dr. J.M. Gelejinse and colleagues also found a significant inverse correlation between long-term, inadequate vitamin K2 intake and aortic calcification. While additional research needs to be done, it looks like maintaining adequate vitamin K levels can help prevent arteriosclerosis and the serious cardiovascular events it can precipitate.

# Vitamin K and Bone Health

Scientists are increasingly recognizing the critical role that vitamin K plays in building strong bones and maintaining bone health. In fact, three proteins that the body uses to form bone tissue—osteocalcin, anticoagulant protein S and matrix gla protein—cannot be activated without sufficient blood levels of vitamin K. Specifically, vitamin K assists in deposition of calcium, magnesium and phosphorus in the bone matrix. Studies have shown that elderly people with low vitamin K intake have suboptimal bone density and are at an increased risk of osteoporosis. Additional evidence from several important clinical trials reveals that vitamin K supplementation—in cases of deficiency—can decrease loss of bone density and overall fracture rates. A 1998 study of postmenopausal women who ate one or more servings of lettuce a day (lettuce is a good source of vitamin K) were 45 percent less likely to have a hip fracture than women who ate one serving or less of lettuce per week.

Another study compared the effects of vitamin K2 on bone mineral density to the effects of estrogen replacement therapy and vitamin D3 supplementation. Researchers divided 72 healthy postmenopausal women into four groups. Women in each group received one of four treatments: a placebo; a vitamin D supplement; hormone replacement therapy; or 45 milligrams per day of supplemental vitamin K2. At baseline and after six and 12 months of treatment, scientists measured bone mineral density in all four groups. They found that the women in the vitamin K and vitamin D groups had significantly less bone loss than the women in the placebo and hormone replacement therapy groups.

# Safety

Nutrition experts consider vitamin K to be safe at recommended dosages. No tolerable upper intake level has been set, and vitamin K deficiencies are quite rare. Because vitamin K is a fat-soluble vitamin and excess amounts remain in the body, consumption above the recommended daily intake levels is not recommended and may cause toxicity.

# Drug/Supplement Interactions

Individuals who are taking antibiotics, anticoagulant/antiplatelet drugs, doxorubicin, laxatives, high doses of vitamin E, weight-loss medications or warfarin (Coumadin) should consult with their physician before taking vitamin K supplements. Additionally, anyone on a daily aspirin regimen to help prevent cardiovascular disease should check with a health care professional before taking vitamin K supplements.

## VITAMIN K FAST FACTS

**Uses and Benefits:** Vitamin K is essential for healthy blood clotting and can help prevent infant hemorrhagic disease. Vitamin K also may support healthy bone mineralization and play a minor role in preventing atherosclerosis.

**Sources:** Dark leafy green vegetables such as spinach, broccoli and kale are rich sources of vitamin K, as are vegetable oils such as canola oil, olive oil, cottonseed oil and soybean oil. Some other fruits, nuts and vegetables contain small amounts of vitamin K.

**Special Considerations:** Vitamin K is generally considered safe, and there is no set tolerable upper intake. Consult with your physician before taking vitamin K supplements if you take aspirin (for your heart), antibiotics, anticoagulants, doxorubicin, laxatives, high doses of vitamin E, weight-loss medications or warfarin (Coumadin).

# Selected References

## Alpha Lipoic Acid

Baur, A. et al. 1991. "Alpha-lipoic acid is an effective inhibitor of human immuno-deficiency virus (HIV-1) replication." *Klin Wochenschr* 69(15): 722–24.

Estrade, D.E. and H.S. Ewart. 1996. "Stimulation of glucose uptake by the natural coenzyme lipoic acid/thioctic acid: participation of elements of the insulin signaling pathway." *Diabetes* 45(12): 1798–1804.

Nagamatsu, M. et al. 1995. "Lipoic acid improves nerve blood flow, reduces oxidative stress, and improves distal nerve conduction in experimental diabetic neuropathy." *Diabetes Care* l18(8): 1160–67.

Packer, L. 1998. "Alpha-lipoic acid: a metabolic antioxidant which regulates NF-kappa B signal transduction and protects against oxidative injury." *Drug Metabolism Review* 30(2): 245–75.

Packer, L. 1996. "Alpha-lipoic acid: the metabolic antioxidant." *Free Radical Biology and Medicine* 20(4): 626–26.

Panigrahi, M. et al. 1996. "Alpha lipoic acid protects against reperfusion injury following cerebral ischemia in rats." *Brain Research* 717(1–2): 184–88.

Ziegler, D. et al. 1999. "Treatment of symptomatic diabetic polyneuropathy with the antioxidant alpha-lipoic acid: a 7-month multicenter randomized controlled trial (ALADIN III Study). ALADIN III Study Group. Alpha-Lipoic Acid in Diabetic Neuropathy." *Diabetes Care* 22(8): 1296–301.

Ziegler, D. et al. 1995. "Treatment of symptomatic diabetic peripheral neuropathy with the antioxidant alpha-lipoic acid. A 3-week multicentre randomized controlled trial (ALADIN Study)." *Diabetologia* 38(12): 1425–33.

Ziegler, D. and H. Schatz. 1997. "Effects of treatment with the antioxidant alpha-lipoic acid on cardiac autonomic neuropathy in NIDDM patients. A 4-month randomized controlled multicenter trial (DEKAN Study)." *Diabetes Care* 20(3): 369–73.

## Antioxidants

Bliss, R.M. 2007. "Nutrition and brain function: food for the aging mind." *Agricultural Research* 55(7): 8–13.

Brody, J.E. 1994. "Scientist at work: Bruce N. Ames; strong views on origins of cancer." *New York Times*, July 5.

Pokorny, J. et al., eds. 2001. *Antioxidants in Food: Practical Applications*. Cambridge, England: Woodhead Publishing Limited.

USDA Agricultural Research Service. 1999. "Can foods forestall aging?" *Agricultural Research* 47(2): 14–17.

**B Vitamins**

Bailey, L.B. 1998. "Dietary reference intakes for folate: the debut of dietary folate equivalents." *Nutrition Reviews* 56(10): 294–99.

Bailey, L.B. and J.F. Gregory 3rd. 1999. "Folate metabolism and requirements." *Journal of Nutrition* 129(4): 779–82.

Benton, D. et al. 1995. "The impact of long-term vitamin supplementation on cognitive functioning." *Psychopharmacology* 117(3): 298–305.

Brody, T. 1999. *Nutritional Biochemistry*, 2nd ed. San Diego, CA: Academic Press.

Canner, P.L. et al. 1986. "Fifteen year mortality in Coronary Drug Project patients: long-term benefit with niacin." *Journal of the American College of Cardiology* 8(6): 1245–55.

Centers for Disease Control and Prevention. 2004. "Spina bifida and anencephaly before and after folic acid mandate—United States, 1995–1996 and 1999–2000. *MMWR* 53(17): 362–65.

Coggeshall, J.C. et al. 1985. "Biotin status and plasma glucose levels in diabetics." *Annals of the New York Academy of Sciences* 447:389–92.

Cumming, R.G. et al. 2000. "Diet and cataract: the Blue Mountains Eye Study." *Ophthalmology* 107(3): 450–56.

Gaddi, A. et al. "Controlled evaluation of pantethine, a natural hypolipidemic compound, in patients with different forms of hyperlipoproteinemia." *Atherosclerosis* 50(1): 73–83.

Jacques, P.F. et al. 2005. "Long-term nutrient intake and 5-year change in nuclear lens opacities." *Archives of Ophthalmology* 123(4): 517–26.

Keniston, R.C. et al. 1997. "Vitamin B6, vitamin C, and carpal tunnel syndrome. A cross-sectional study of 441 adults" *Journal of Occupational and Environmental Medicine* 39(10): 949–59.

Kim, Y.I. et al. 2001. "Effects of folate supplementation on two provisional molecular markers of colon cancer: a prospective, randomized trial." *American Journal of Gastroenterology* 96(1): 184–95.

Lajous, M. et al. 2006. "Folate, vitamin B(6), and vitamin B(12) intake and the risk of breast cancer among Mexican women." *Cancer Epidemiology, Biomarkers & Prevention* 15(3): 443–48.

Lajous, M. et al. 2006. "Folate, vitamin B12 and postmenopausal breast cancer in a prospective study of French women." *Cancer Causes & Control* 17(9): 1209–13.

Leske, M.C. et al. 1995. "Biochemical factors in the lens opacities. Case-control study. The Lens Opacities Case-Control Study Group." *Archives of Ophthalmology* 113(9): 1113–19.

Maebashi, M. et al. 1993. "Therapeutic evaluation of the effect of biotin on hyperglycemia in patients with non-insulin dependent diabetes mellitus." *Journal of Clinical Biochemistry and Nutrition* 14(3): 211–18.

Martin, P.R. et al. 2003. "The role of thiamine deficiency in alcoholic brain disease." *Alcoholic Research & Health* 27(2): 134–42.

No author listed. 1998. "Lowering blood homocysteine with folic acid based supplements: meta-analysis of randomised trials. Homocysteine Lowering Trialists' Collaboration." *BMJ* 316(7135): 894–98.

Penninx, B.W. et al. 2000. "Vitamin B(12) deficiency and depression in physically disabled older women: epidemiologic evidence from the Women's Health and Aging Study." *American Journal of Psychiatry* 157(5): 715–21.

Powers, H.J. 1999. "Current knowledge concerning optimum nutritional status of riboflavin, niacin and pyridoxine." *Proceedings of the Nutrition Society* 58(2): 435–40.

Quinlivan, E.P. et al. 2002. "Importance of both folic acid and vitamin B12 in reduction of risk of vascular disease." *Lancet* 359(9302): 227–28.

Riggs, K.M. et al. 1996. "Relations of vitamin B-12, vitamin B-6, folate, and homocysteine to cognitive performance in the Normative Aging Study." *American Journal of Clinical Nutrition* 63(3): 306–14.

Rimm, E.B. et al. 1998. "Folate and vitamin B6 from diet and supplements in relation to risk of coronary heart disease among women." *JAMA* 279(5): 359–64.

Sahakian, V. et al. 1991. "Vitamin B6 is effective therapy for nausea and vomiting of pregnancy: a randomized, double-blind placebo-controlled study." *Obstetrics and Gynecology* 78(1): 33–36.

Sándor, P.S. et al. 2000. "Prophylactic treatment of migraine with beta-blockers and riboflavin: differential effects on the intensity dependence of auditory evoked cortical potentials." *Headache* 40(1): 30–35.

Schoenen, J. et al. 1998. "Effectiveness of high-dose riboflavin in migraine prophylaxis. A randomized controlled trial." *Neurology* 50(2): 466–70.

Selhub, J. et al. 2000. "B vitamins, homocysteine, and neurocognitive function in the elderly." *American Journal of Clinical Nutrition* 71(2): 614S–620S.

Shrubsole, M.J. et al. 2001. "Dietary folate intake and breast cancer risk: results from the Shanghai Breast Cancer Study." *Cancer Research* 61(19): 7136–41.

Smidt, L.J. et al. 1991. "Influence of thiamin supplementation on the health and general well-being of an elderly Irish population with marginal thiamin deficiency." *Journal of Gerontology* 46(1): M16–22.

Tahiliani, A.G. and C.J. Beinlich. 1991. "Pantothenic acid in health and disease." *Vitamins and Hormones* 146:165–228.

Tiemeier, H. et al. 2002. "Vitamin B12, folate, and homocysteine in depression: the Rotterdam Study."*American Journal of Psychiatry* 159(12): 2099–101.

Voutilainen, S. et al. 2001. "Low dietary folate intake is associated with an excess incidence of acute coronary events: the Kuopio Ischemic Heart Disease Risk Factor Study." *Circulation* 103(22): 2674–80.

Vutyavanich, T. et al. 1995. "Pyridoxine for nausea and vomiting of pregnancy: a randomized, double-blind, placebo-controlled trial." *American Journal of Obstetrics and Gynecology* 173(3 Pt 1): 881–84.

Wang, H.X. et al. "Vitamin B(12) and folate in relation to the development of Alzheimer's disease." *Neurology* 56(9): 1188–94.

Weimann, B.I. and D. Hermann. 1999. "Studies on wound healing: effects of calcium D-pantothenate on the migration, proliferation and protein synthesis of human dermal fibroblasts in culture." *International Journal for Vitamin and Nutrition Research* 69(2): 113–19.

Wink, J. et al. 2002. "Effect of very-low-dose niacin on high-density lipoprotein in patients undergoing long-term statin therapy." *American Heart Journal* 143(3): 514–18.

Zhang, S. et al. 1999. "A prospective study of folate intake and the risk of breast cancer." *JAMA* 281(17): 1632–37.

**Carnitine**

Atar, D. et al. 1997. "Carnitine—from cellular mechanisms to potential clinical applications in heart disease." *European Journal of Clinical Investigation* 27(12): 973–76.

Benvenga, S. and R.M. Ruggeri. 2001. "Usefulness of L-carnitine, a naturally occurring peripheral antagonist of thyroid hormone action, in iatrogenic hyperthyroidism: a randomized, double-blind, placebo-controlled clinical trial." *Journal of Clinical Endocrinology and Metabolism* 86(8): 3579–94.

Cruciani, R.A. et al. 2004. "L-carnitine supplementation for the treatment of fatigue and depressed mood in cancer patients with carnitine deficiency: a preliminary analysis." *Annals of the New York Academy of Sciences* 1033:168–76.

Garolla, A. et al. 2005. "Oral carnitine supplementation increases sperm motility in asthenozoospermic men with normal sperm phospholipid hydroperoxide glutathione peroxidase levels." *Fertility and Sterility* 83(2): 355–61.

Hiatt, W.R. and J.G. Regensteiner. 2001. "Propionyl-L-carnitine improves exercise performance and functional status in patients with claudication." *American Journal of Medicine* 110(8): 616–22.

Lenzi, A. et al. 2005. "A placebo-controlled double-blind randomized trial of the use of combined l-carnitine and l-acetyl-carnitine treatment in men with asthenozoospermia." *Fertility and Sterility* 84(3): 662–71.

Ng, C.M. et al. 2005. "The role of carnitine in the male reproductive system." *Annals of the New York Academy of Sciences* 1033:177–88.

Pauly, D.F. and C.J. Pepine. 2003. "The role of carnitine in myocardial dysfunction." *American Journal of Kidney Disorders* 41(4 Suppl 4): S35–43.

Plioplys, A.V. and S. Plioplys. 1997. "Amantadine and L-carnitine treatment of chronic fatigue syndrome." *Neuropsychobiology* 35(1): 16–23.

Rizos, I. and W.R. Hiatt. 2000. "Three-year survival of patients with heart failure caused by dilated cardiomyopathy and L-carnitine administration." *American Heart Journal* 139(2 Pt 3): S120–23.

Sano, M. et al. 1992. "Double-blind parallel design pilot study of acetyl levocarnitine in patients with Alzheimer's disease." *Archives of Neurology* 49(11):1137–41.

Singh, R.B. et al. 1996. "A randomised, double-blind, placebo-controlled trial of L-carnitine in suspected acute myocardial infarction." *Postgraduate Medical Journal* 72(843): 45–50.

Spagnoli, A. et al. 1991. "Long-term acetyl-L-carnitine treatment in Alzheimer's disease." *Neurology* 41(11): 1726–32.

**Cinnamon**

Blumenthal, M. 2000. *Herbal Medicine: Expanded Commission E Monographs.* Austin, TX: American Botanical Council.

Chase, C.K. and C.E. McQueen. 2007. "Cinnamon in diabetes mellitus." *American Journal of Health-System Pharmacy* 64(10): 1033–35.

Fabio, A. et al. 2007. "Screening of the antibacterial effects of a variety of essential oils on microorganisms responsible for respiratory infections." *Phytotherapy Research* 21(4): 374–77.

Hlebowicz, J. et al. 2007. "Effect of cinnamon on postprandial blood glucose, gastric emptying, and satiety in healthy subjects." *American Journal of Clinical Nutrition* 85(6): 1552–56.

Hoque, M.M. et al. 2007. "Antimicrobial activity of cloves and cinnamon extracts against food-borne pathogens and spoilage bacteria, and inactivation of *Listeria monocytogenes* in ground chicken meat with their essential oils." *Journal of Food Science and Technology* 72:9–21.

Kaul, P.N. et al. 2003. "Volatile constituents of essential oils isolated from different parts of cinnamon (*Cinnamomum zeylanicum* Blume)." *Journal of the Science of Food and Agriculture* 83(1): 53–55.

Khan, A. et al. 2003. "Cinnamon improves glucose and lipids of people with type 2 diabetes." *Diabetes Care* 26(12): 3215–18.

Mang, B. et al. 2006. "Effects of a cinnamon extract on plasma glucose, HbA, and serum lipids in diabetes mellitus type 2." *European Journal of Clinical Investigation* 36 (5): 340–44.

Osborne, T.D. 2000. *A Taste of Paradise: Cinnamon.* James Ford Bell Library, University of Minnesota. http://bell.lib.umn. edu/Products/cinnamon. html.

Oussalah, M. et al. 2006. "Antimicrobial effects of selected plant essential oils on the growth of a *Pseudomonas putida* strain isolated from meat." *Meat Science* 73(2): 236–44.

Pham, A.Q. et al. 2007. "Cinnamon supplementation in patients with type 2 diabetes mellitus." *Pharmacotherapy* 27(4): 595–99.

Ravindran, P.N. et al. 2003. *Cinnamon and Cassia: The Genus Cinnamomum.* Boca Raton, FL: CRC Press.

Quale, J.M. et al. 1996. "In vitro activity of Cinnamomum zeylanicum against azole resistant and sensitive Candida species and a pilot study of cinnamon for oral candidiasis." *American Journal of Chinese Medicine* 24(2): 103–10.

Ravishankar, S. et al. 2008. "Plant-derived compounds inactivate antibiotic-resistant *Campylobacter jejuni* strains." *Journal of Food Protection* 71(6): 1145–49.

Raudenbush, B. 2004. "Effects of peppermint on enhancing mental performance and cognitive functioning, pain threshold and tolerance, digestion and digestive processes, and athletic performance." Prepared exclusively for the Sense of Smell Institute—the research and education division of the Fragrance Foundation.

Subash Babu, P. et al. 2007. "Cinnamaldehyde—a potential antidiabetic agent." *Phytomedicine* 14(1): 15–22.

Tabak, M. et al. 1999. "Cinnamon extracts' inhibitory effect on *Helicobacter pylori*." *Journal of Ethnopharmacology* 67(3): 269–77.

Valero, M. and M.C. Salmerón. 2003. "Antibacterial activity of 11 essential oils against Bacillus cereus in tyndallized carrot broth." *International Journal of Food Microbiology* 85(1–2): 73–81.

Verspohl, E.J. et al. 2005. "Antidiabetic effect of *Cinnamomum cassia* and *Cinnamomum zeylanicum* in vivo and in vitro." *Phytotherapy Research* 19(3): 203–06.

Ziegenfuss, T.N. et al. 2006. "Effects of a water-soluble cinnamon extract on body composition and features of the metabolic syndrome in pre-diabetic men and women." *Journal of the International Society of Sport Nutrition* 28(3): 45–53.

## CoQ10

Baggio, E. et al. 1994. "Italian multicenter study on the safety and efficacy of coenzyme Q10 as adjunctive therapy in heart failure. CoQ10 Drug Surveillance Investigators." *Molecular Aspects of Medicine* 15(Suppl): S287–94.

Bonakdar, R.A. and E. Guarneri. "Coenzyme Q10." *American Family Physician.* 72(6): 1065–70.

Dhanasekaran, M. and J. Ren. 2005. "The emerging role of coenzyme Q-10 in aging, neurodegeneration, cardiovascular disease, cancer and diabetes mellitus." *Current Neurovascular Research* 2(5): 447–59.

Fonorow, O.R. 2006. "CoQ10 and statins: the vitamin C connection." *Townsend Letter* (online). http://www.townsendletter.com/FebMar2006/coq100206.htm.

Honda, K. et al. 2007. "Thirteen-week repeated dose of oral toxicity study of coenzyme Q10 in rats." *Journal of Toxicological Sciences* 32(4): 437–48.

Ito, T. et al. 2006. "Potentiated effects of coenzyme Q10 complex supplement on Endurance and stamina of middle aged men." *Pharmacometrics* 71(1–2): 29–35.

Jeejeebhoy, F. et al. 2002. "Nutritional supplementation with MyoVive repletes essential cardiac myocyte nutrients and reduces left ventricular size in patients with left ventricular dysfunction." *American Heart Journal* 143(6): 1092–100.

Shults, C.W. et al. 2002. "Effects of coenzyme Q10 in early Parkinson disease: evidence of slowing of the functional decline." *Archives of Neurology* 59(10): 1541–50.

Soja, A.M. and S.A Mortenson. 1997. "Treatment of congestive heart failure with coenzyme Q10 illuminated by meta-analyses of clinical trials." *Molecular Aspects of Medicine* 18(Suppl): S159–68.

Shekelle, P. et al. 2003. "Effect of supplemental antioxidants vitamin C, vitamin E, and coenzyme Q10 for the prevention and treatment of cardiovascular disease. Evidence Report/Technology Assessment No. 83. Rockville, MD: Agency for Healthcare Research and Quality.

**Cranberries**

Ackerson, A.D. 2005. "Cranberry (*Vaccinium macrocarpon*)." *Better Nutrition* 67(5): 12.

American Gastroenterological Association. "Peptic Ulcer Disease." AGA Patient Center. and "Peptic Ulcer Disease and *H. Pylori*." http://www.gastro.org/wmspage.cfm?parm1=5686.

American Physiological Society. 2005. Press release: "Cranberry juice modulates atherosclerotic vascular dysfunction." April 3.

Barnes, N.B. et al. 2002. "Consumers, cranberries, and cures: what consumers know about the health benefits of cranberries." Slade's Ferry Bank Center for Business Research.

Burger, O. et al. 2000. "A high molecular mass constituent of cranberry juice inhibits *Helicobacter pylori* adhesion to human gastric mucus." *FEMS Immunology and Medical Microbiology* 29(4): 295–301.

Chu, Y.F. amd R.H. Liu. 2005. "Cranberries inhibit LDL oxidation and induce LDL receptor expression in hepatocytes." *Life Sciences* 77(15): 1892–901.

Cranberry Institute. "Cranberry health update: cranberry nutritional composition." http://cranberryinstitute.org/news/nutritional.pdf.

Fleet, J.C. 1994. "New support for a folk remedy: cranberry juice reduces bacteriuria and pyuria in elderly women." *Nutrition Review* 52(5): 168–70.

Ferguson, P.J. et al. 2004. "Flavonoid fraction from cranberry extract inhibits proliferation of human tumor cell lines." *Journal of Nutrition* 134(6): 1529–35.

Gettmann, M.T. et al. 2005. "Effect of cranberry juice consumption on urinary stone risk factors." *Journal of Urology* 174(2): 590–94.

Howell, A.B. et al. 2005. "A-type cranberry proanthocyanidins and uropathogenic bacterial anti-adhesion activity." *Phytochemistry* 66(18): 2281–91.

Jepson, R.G. et al. 2005. "Cranberries for preventing urinary tract infections." *Journal of Urology* 173(1): 111–12.

Kurutas, E.B. et al. 2005. "The effects of oxidative stress in urinary tract infection." *Mediators of Inflammation* 4:242–44.

Leahy, M. 2002. "Latest developments in cranberry health research." *Pharmaceutical Biology* 40 (suppl): 50–54.

Lin, Y.T. et al. 2005. "Inhibition of *Helicobacter pylori* and associated urease by oregano and cranberry phytochemical synergies." *Applied and Environmental Microbiology* 71(12): 8558–64.

Lynch, D.M. 2004. "Cranberry for prevention of urinary tract infections." *American Family Physician* 70 (11): 2175–77.

National Kidney and Urologic Disease Information Clearinghouse (NKUDIC) "Urinary tract infections in adults." http://kidney.niddk.nih.gov/kudiseases/pubs/utiadult/.

Puupponin-Pimia, R. et al. 2005. "Bioactive berry compounds—novel tools against human pathogens." *Applied Microbiology and Biotechnology* 67 (1): 8–18.

Reed, J. 2002. "Cranberry flavonoids, atherosclerosis, and cardiovascular health." *Critical Reviews in Food Science Nutrition* 42 (3 suppl) 301–16.

Schardt, D. 2005. "Berry berry good?" *Nutrition Action Health Letter* 32(5): 8–9.

Schieszer, J. 2005. "Cranberry products may prevent UTIs: ingestion of cranberry capsules suppresses three common pathogens in urine specimens." *Renal Urology News* 4(10): 11.

Schmidt, D.R. and A.E. Sobata. 1988. "Examination of the anti-adherence activity of cranberry juice on urinary and nonurinary bacterial isolates." *Microbios* 55(224–225): 173–81.

Seeram, N.P. et al. 2004. "Total cranberry extract versus its phytochemical constituents: antiproliferative and synergistic effects against human tumor cell lines," *Journal of Agriculture and Food Chem*istry 52(9): 2512–17.

Shmuely, H. et al. 2004. "Susceptibility of *Helicobacter pylori* isolates to the antiadhesion activity of a high-molecular-weight constituent of cranberry." *Diagnostic Microbiology and Infectious Diseases* 50(4): 231–35.

Sifton, D.W., ed. 2003. "Putting an end to urinary tract infections." In *PDR Family Guide to Women's Health and Prescription Drugs*. Montvale, NJ: Medical Economics Co.

UMass Cranberry Station. 2006. "Natural history of the American cranberry." University of Massachusetts Amherst. http://www.umass.edu/cranberry/cranberry/seasons.shtml.

University of Massachusetts Dartmouth. 2006. Press release: "New study finds cranberry compounds block cancer: first study to confirm cranberry proanthocyanidins inhibit growth of tumor cells." *PR Newswire* January 25.

Weiss, E.I. et al. 2002. "Inhibitory effect of a high-molecular-weight constituent of cranberry on adhesion of oral bacteria." *Critical Reviews in Food Science and Nutrition* 42(3 suppl): 285–92.

Weiss, E.L. et al. 1998. "Inhibiting interspecies coaggregation of plaque bacteria with a cranberry juice constituent." *Journal of the American Dental Association* 129(12): 1719–23.

Xiaojun, Y. et al. 2002. "Antioxidant activities and antitumor screening of extracts from cranberry fruit." *Journal of Agricultural and Food Chemistry* 50(21): 5844–49.

Zhang, L. et al. 2005. "Efficacy of cranberry juice on *Helicobacter pylori* infection: a double-blind, randomized placebo-controlled trial." *Helicobacter* 10(2): 139–45.

**Grape Seed Extract and Resveratrol**

Block, W. 2005. "Resveratrol and quercetin—puzzling gifts of nature." *Life Enhancement*. http://www.life-enhancement.com/article_template.asp?ID=1098.

Carluccio, M.A. et al. 2003. "Olive oil and red wine antioxidant polyphenols inhibit endothelial activation: antiatherogenic properties of Mediterranean diet phytochemicals." *Arteriosclerosis, Thrombosis, and Vascular Biology* 23(4): 622–29.

Corbé, C. et al. 1988. "Light vision and chorioretinal circulation. Study of the effect of procyanidolic oligomers (endotelon) [article in French]." *Journal français d'ophtalmologie* 11(5): 453–60.

de Santi, C. et al. 2000. "Glucuronidation of resveratrol, a natural product present in grape and wine, in the human liver." *Xenobiotica* 30(11): 1047–54.

Linus Pauling Institute Micronutrient Information Center. "Resveratrol." Oregon State University. http://lpi.oregonstate.edu/infocenter/phytochemicals/resveratrol/.

Mnjoyan, Z.H. and K. Fujise. 2003. "Profound negative effects of resveratrol on vascular smooth muscle cells: a role of p53-p21(WAF1/CIP1) pathway." *Biochemical & Biophysical Research Communications* 311(2): 546–52.

Ong, D. 2006. "Grape seed extract may have blood pressure reducing qualities." *Medical News Today.* http://www.medicalnewstoday.com/articles/40341.php.

Pace-Asciak, C.R. et al. 1995. "The red wine phenolics trans-resveratrol and quercetin block human platelet aggregation and eicosanoid synthesis: implications for protection against coronary heart disease." *Clinica Chimica Acta* 235(2): 207–19.

Preuss, H.G. et al. 2000. "Effects of niacin-bound chromium and grape seed proanthocyanidin extract on the lipid profile of hypercholesterolemic subjects: a pilot study." *Journal of Medicine* 31(5–6): 227–46.

Stein, J.H. et al. 1999. "Purple grape juice improves endothelial function and reduces the susceptibility of LDL cholesterol to oxidation in patients with coronary artery disease." *Circulation* 100:1050–55.

Vogels, N. et al. 2004. "The effect of grape-seed extract on 24 h energy intake in humans." *European Journal of Clinical Nutrition* 58(4): 667–73.

Walle, T. et al. 2004. "High absorption but very low bioavailability of oral resveratrol in humans." *Drug Metabolism and Disposition* 12:1377–82.

Wallerath, T. et al. 2002. "Resveratrol, a polyphenolic phytoalexin present in red wine, enhances expression and activity of endothelial nitric oxide synthase." *Circulation* 106(13): 1652–58.

Wenzel, E. and V. Somoza. 2005. "Metabolism and bioavailability of trans-resveratrol." *Molecular Nutrition & Food Research* 49(5): 472–81.

**Green Tea**

Abe, Y. et al. 1995. "Effect of green tea rich in gamma-aminobutyric acid on blood pressure of Dahl salt-sensitive rats." *American Journal of Hypertension* 8(1): 74–79.

Amarowicz, R. et al. 2005. "Antioxidant and antibacterial properties of extracts of green tea polyphenols." In Shahidi, F. and C.T. Ho, eds. *Phenolic Compounds in Foods and Natural Health Products.* Washington, DC: American Chemical Society: 94–106.

Blumenthal, M. 2000. *Herbal Medicine: Expanded Edition E Monographs.* Newton, Mass.: Integrative Medicine.

Chung, F.L. et al. 2003. "Tea and cancer prevention: studies in animals and humans." *Journal of Nutrition* 133(10): 3268S–74S.

Cooper, R. et al. 2005. "Medicinal benefits of green tea: part I. Review of non-cancer health benefits." *Journal of Alternative and Complementary Medicine* 11(3): 521–28.

Gradišar, H. et al. 2007. "Green tea catechins inhibit bacterial DNA gyrase by interaction with its ATP binding site." *Journal of Medicinal Chemistry* 50(2): 264–71.

Hamilton-Miller, J.M. 2001. "Anti-cariogenic properties of tea (*Camellia sinensis*)." *Journal of Medical Microbiology* 50(4): 299–302.

Hodgson, J.M. et al. 2000. "Acute effects of ingestion of green and black tea on lipoprotein oxidation." *American Journal of Clinical Nutrition* 71(5): 1103–07.

Kono, S. et al. 1992. "Green tea consumption and serum lipid profiles: a cross-sectional study in northern Kyushu, Japan." *Preventive Medicine* 21(4): 526–31.

Kuriyama, S. et al. 2006. "Green tea consumption and cognitive function: a cross-sectional study from the tsurugaya project." *American Journal of Clinical Nutrition* 83(2): 355–61.

Mandel, S. and M.B. Youdim. 2004. "Catechin polyphenols: neurodegeneration and neuroprotection in neurodegenerative diseases." *Free Radical Biology & Medicine* 37(3): 304–17.

*Natural Medicine's Comprehensive Database*. 2002. Stockton, CA: Therapeutic Research Facility.

Riemersma, R.A. et al. 2001. "Tea flavonoids and cardiovascular health." *QJM* 94(5): 277–82.

Rietveldt, A. and S. Wiseman. 2003. "Antioxidant effects of tea: evidence from human clinical trials." *Journal of Nutrition* 133(10): 3285S–92S.

Scalbert, A. et al. 2005. "Polyphenols: antioxidants and beyond." *American Journal of Clinical Nutrition* 81(Suppl): 215S–17S.

Siddiqui, I.A. et al. 2004. "Antioxidants of the beverage tea in the promotion of human health." *Antioxidant & Redox Signaling* 6(3): 571–82.

Song, J.M. et al. 2005. "Antiviral effect of catechins in green tea on influenza." *Antiviral Research* 68(2): 66–74.

Unno, T. et al. 1996. "Analysis of epigallocatechin gallate in human serum obtained after ingesting green tea." *Bioscience, Biotechnology, and Biochemistry* 60(12): 2066–68.

Xu, J. et al. 2008. "Green tea extract and its major component epigallocatechin gallate inhibits hepatitis B virus in vitro." *Antiviral Research* 78(3): 242–49.

Yang, T.T. and M.W. Koo. 1997. "Hypocholesterolemic effects of Chinese tea." *Pharmacological Research* 35(6): 505–12.

Yang, Y.C. et al. 2004. "Protective effect of habitual tea consumption on hypertension." *Archives of Internal Medicine* 164(14): 1534–40.

**Multivitamin/Multi-Mineral Supplements**

Brody, T. 1999. *Nutritional Biochemistry*, 2nd ed. San Diego, CA: Academic Press.

Cooperman, T. et al, eds. 2003. *ConsumerLab.com's Guide to Buying Vitamins and Supplements*. White Plains, NY: ConsumerLab.com Publications.

Dunne, L.J. 2002. *Nutrition Almanac*, 5th ed. New York: McGraw-Hill.

Fragakis, A.S. and C. Thompson. 2007. *The Health Professional's Guide to Popular Dietary Supplements*, 3rd ed. Chicago, IL: American Dietetic Association.

Griffith, H.W. 1988. *Complete Guide to Vitamins, Minerals, and Supplements*. Tucson, AZ: Fisher Books.

MacWilliam, L. 2003. *Comparative Guide to Nutritional Supplements*. Vernon, British Columbia: Northern Dimensions.

Murray, M.T. 1996 *Encyclopedia of Nutritional Supplements*. New York: Three Rivers.

Shils, M.E. et al. 2006. *Modern Nutrition in Health and Disease*, 3rd ed. Baltimore: Lippincott Williams & Wilkins.

Talbott, S.M. 2003. *A Guide to Understanding Dietary Supplements*. New York: Haworth.

Webb, G. 2006. *Dietary Supplements and Functional Foods*. Oxford, England: Blackwell.

Zimmermann, M. 2001. *Pocket Guide to Micronutrients in Health and Disease*. New York: Thieme.

**Nattokinase**

Amano Enzyme, Inc. 2002. "Natto—traditional Japanese fermented soy beans with recently discovered health benefits and novel industrial applications." *Enzyme Wave* 3:2–4.

eMedicine. "Toxicity, warfarin and superwarfarins." WebMD. http://www. emedicine.com/emerg/topic872.htm.

Fujita, M. et al. 1995. "Thrombolytic effect of nattokinase on a chemically induced thrombosis model in rat." *Biological & Pharmaceutical Bulletin* 18(10): 1387–91.

Kraaijenhagen, R.A. and H.R. Büller. 2001. "Travel and risk of venous thrombosis." *Lancet* 357(9255): 554.

Maruyama, M. and H. Sumi, eds.. 1995. "Effect of natto diet on blood pressure." In *Basic Clinical Aspects of Japanese Traditional Food*. Japan Technology Transfer Association. 1–3.

Nishimura, K. et al. 1994. "Natto diet was apparently effective in a case of incipient central retinal vein occlusion." *Japanese Review of Clinical Ophthalmology* 88:1381-85.

Sumi, H. et al. 2005. "A novel fibrinolytic enzyme (nattokinase) in the vegetable cheese Natto; a typical and popular soybean food in the Japanese diet." *Cellular and Molecular Life Sciences* 43(10): 1110–11.

Sumi, H. et al. 1990. "Enhancement of the fibrinolytic activity in plasma by oral administration of nattokinase." *Acta Haematologica* 84(3): 139–43.

Suzuki, Y. et al. 2003. "Dietary supplementation with fermented soybeans suppresses intimal thickening." *Nutrition* 19(3): 261–64.

Suzuki, Y. et al. 2003. "Dietary supplementation of fermented soybean, natto, suppresses intimal thickening and modulates the lysis of mural thrombi after endothelial injury in rat femoral artery." *Life Sciences* 73(10) 1289–98.

**Natural Sweeteners**

AAPD Council on Clinical Affairs. 2006. "Policy on the use of xylitol in caries prevention." American Academy of Pediatric Dentistry. http://www.aapd. org/media/Policies_Guidelines/P_Xylitol.pdf.

Dhingra, R. et al. 2007. "Soft drink consumption and risk of developing cardiometabolic risk factors and the metabolic syndrome in middle aged adults in the community." *Circulation* 116(5): 480–488.

Gold, A. 2008. "Food conscious: just a spoonful of agave syrup." SF Gate. http://www.sfgate.com/cgi-bin/article.cgi?f=/c/a/2008/06/18/FDEJ116TOH.DTL

Gross, L.S. et al. 2004. "Increased consumption of refined carbohydrates and the epidemic of type 2 diabetes in the United States: an ecologic assessment." *American Journal of Clinical Nutrition* 79(5): 774–79.

Higdon, J. "Glycemic index and glycemic load." Linus Pauling Institute. http://lpi.oregonstate.edu/infocenter/foods/grains/gigl.html.

International Food Information Council. 2008. "Sugar alcohols fact sheet."

http://www.ific.org/publications/factsheets/sugaralcoholfs.cfm.

Jones, J.L. "Stevia: toxic or tasty." About.com Holistic Healing. http://healing. about.com/cs/uc_directory/a/uc_stevia_jones.htm.

Konoshima, T. and M. Takasaki. 2002. "Cancer-chemopreventive effects of natural sweeteners and related compounds." *Pure and Applied Chemistry* 74(7): 1309–1316.

Lim, U. et al. 2006. "Consumption of aspartame-containing beverages and incidence of hematopoietic and brain malignancies." *Cancer Epidemiology, Biomarkers & Prevention* 15(9): 1654–59.

Mäkinen, K.K. et al. 1995. "Xylitol chewing gum and caries rates: a 40-month cohort study." *Journal of Dental Research* 74(12): 1904–13.

Mann, J. 2004. "Free sugars and human health: sufficient evidence for action?" *Lancet* 363(9414): 1068–70.

Mardis, A.L. 2001. "Current knowledge of the health effects of sugar intake." *Family Economics and Nutrition Review* 13(1): 87–91.

Nestle, M. 2006. *What to Eat*. New York: North Point Press.

Schardt, D. 2000. "Stevia: a bittersweet tale." *Nutrition Action* (April). http:// www.cspinet.org/nah/4_00/stevia.html.

Suzuki, Y.A. et al. 2005. "Triterpene glycosides of Siraitia grosvenori inhibit rat intestinal maltase and suppress the rise in blood glucose level after a single oral administration of maltose in rats." *Journal of Agricultural and Food Chemistry* 53(8): 2941–46.

Swithers, S.E. and T.L. Davidson. 2008. "A role for sweet taste: calorie predictive relations in energy regulation by rats." *Behavioral Neuroscience* 122(1): 161–73.

Takasaki, M. 2003. "Anticarcinogenic activity of natural sweeteners, cucurbitane glycosides, from Momordica grosvenori." *Cancer Letters* 198(1): 37–42.

## Omega-3 Essential Fatty Acids

Bang, H.O. and J. Dyerberg. 1980. "Lipid metabolism and ischemic heart disease in Greenland Eskimos." In Draper, H. ed. *Advances in Nutrition Research*. New York: Plenum. 1–22.

Berquin, I.M. et al. 2007. "Modulation of prostate cancer genetic risk by omega-3 and omega-6 fatty acids." *Journal of Clinical Investigation* 117(7): 1866–75.

Fortin, P.R. et al. 1995. "Validation of a meta-analysis: the effects of fish oil in rheumatoid arthritis." *Journal of Clinical Epidemiology* 48(11): 1379–90.

Freedman, S.D. et al. 2004. "Association of cystic fibrosis with abnormalities in fatty acid metabolism." *New England Journal of Medicine* 350(6): 560–69.

Geelen, A. et al. 2007. "Fish consumption, n-3 fatty acids, and colorectal cancer: a meta-analysis of prospective cohort studies." *American Journal of Epidemiology* 166(10): 1116–25.

Harris, W.S. and C. von Schacky. 2004. "The Omega-3 Index: a new risk factor for death from coronary heart disease?" *Preventive Medicine* 39(1): 212–20.

O'Keefe, J.H. and W.S. Harris. 2000. "From Inuit to implementation: omega-3 fatty acids come of age." *Mayo Clinic Proceedings* 75:607–14.

Richter, W.O. 2003. "Long chain omega-3 fatty acids from fish reduce sudden cardiac death in patients with coronary heart disease." *European Journal of Medical Research* 8(8): 332–36.

Shannon, J. "Erythrocyte fatty acids and breast cancer risk: a case control study in Shanghai, China." *American Journal Clinical Nutrition* 85(4): 1090–97.

Shapiro, J.A. et al. 1996. "Diet and rheumatoid arthritis in women: a possible protective effect of fish consumption." *Epidemiology* 7(3): 256–63.

Simopoulos, A.P. 2002. "The importance of the ratio of omega-6/omega-3 essential fatty acids." *Biomedicine & Pharmacotherapy* 56(8): 365–79.

**Probiotics**

Bertazzoni, M.E. et al. 2000. "Preliminary screening of health-Promoting properties of new *Lactobacillus* strain: in vitro and in vivo." 2000 HEALFO abstracts.

Casas, I.A. and W.J. Dobrogosz. 2000. "Validation of the probiotic concept: *Lactobacillus reuteri* confers broad-spectrum protection against disease in humans and animals." *Microbial Ecology in Health and Disease* 12(4): 247–85.

Collins, D.C. and G.R. Gibson. 1999. "Probiotics, prebiotics and synbiotics: approaches for modulating the microbial ecology of the gut." *American Journal of Clinical Nutrition* 69(5): 1052S–57S.

D'Souza, A.L. et al. 2002. "Probiotics in prevention of antibiotic associated diarrhoea: meta-analysis." *BMJ* 324(7350): 1361.

Elmer, G.W. 2001. "Probiotics: 'living drugs.'" *American Journal of Health-System Pharmacy* 58(12): 1101–09.

Isolauri, E. et al. 2002. "Probiotics: a role in the treatment of intestinal infection and inflammation?" *Gut* 50(Suppl 3): III54–59.

Jiang, T. et al. 1996. "Improvement of lactose digestion in humans by ingestion of unfermented milk containing *Bifidobacterium longum*." *Journal of Dairy Science* 79(5): 750–57.

Kailasapathy, K. and J. Chin. 2000. "Survival and therapeutic potential of probiotic organisms with reference to *Lactobacillus acidophilus* and *Bifidobacterium* spp." *Immunology and Cell Biology* 78(1): 80–88.

Macfarlane, G.T. and J.H. Cummings. 1999. "Probiotics and prebiotics: can regulating the activities of intestinal bacteria benefit health?" *BMJ* 318(7189): 999–1003.

Mattman, L.H. 2001. *Cell Wall Deficient Forms: Stealth Pathogens*, third ed. Boca Raton, FL: CRC Press.

Sartor, R.B. 2005. "Probiotic therapy of intestinal inflammation and infections." *Current Opinion in Gastroenterology* 21(1): 44–50.

Schrezenmeir, J. and M. de Vrese. 2001. "Probiotics, prebiotics and synbiotics—approaching a definition." *American Journal of Clinical Nutrition* 73(2 Suppl): 361S–64S.

Söderholm, J.D. and M.H. Perdue. 2001. "Stress and the gastrointestinal tract II. Stress and intestinal barrier function." *American Journal of Physiology. Gastrointestinal and Liver Physiology* 280(1): G7–G13.

Vanderhoof, J.A. and R.J. Young. 2002. "Current and potential uses of probiotics." *Annals of Allergy, Asthma and Immunology* 93(Suppl 3): S33–S37.

Walker, W.A. and L.C. Duffy. 1998. "Diet and bacterial colonisation: role of probiotics and prebiotics." *Journal of Nutritional Biochemistry* 9(12): 668–75.

Yan, F. and D.B. Polk. 2004. "Commensal bacteria in the gut: learning who our friends are." *Current Opinions in Gastroenterology* 20(6): 565–71.

## Soy

Allison, D.B. et al. 2003. "A novel soy-based meal replacement for weight loss among obese individuals: a randomized controlled clinical trial." *European Journal of Clinical Nutrition* 57(4): 514–22.

Campbell, C.G. et al. 2006. "Effects of soy or milk protein during a high-fat feeding challenge on oxidative stress, inflammation, and lipids in healthy men." *Lipids* 41(3): 257–65.

Divi, R.L. et al. 1997. "Anti-thyroid isoflavones from soybean: isolation, characterization, and mechanisms of action." *Biochemical Pharmacology* 54(10): 1087–96.

Fotsis, T. et al. 1993. "Genistein, a dietary-derived inhibitor of in vitro angiogenesis." *Proceedings of the National Academy of Sciences of the United States of America* 90(7): 2690–2694.

Hooper, L. et al. 2008. "Flavonoids, flavonoid-rich foods, and cardiovascular risk: a metal-analysis of randomized controlled trials." *American Journal of Clinical Nutrition* 88(1): 38–50.

Lichenstein, G.R. et al. 2008. "Bowman-Birk inhibitor concentrate: a novel therapeutic agent for patients with active ulcerative colitis." *Digestive Diseases and Sciences* 53(1): 175–80.

Nelson, H.D. et al. 2006. "Nonhormonal therapies for menopausal hot flashes: systematic review and meta-analysis." *JAMA* 295(17): 2057–71.

Picherit, C. et al. 2000. "Daidzein is more efficient than genistein in preventing ovariectomy-induced bone loss in rats." *Journal of Nutrition* 130(7): 1675–81.

Setchell, K.D. and E. Lydeking-Olsen. 2003. "Dietary phytoestrogens and their effect on bone: evidence from in vitro and in vivo, human observationsl, and dietary intervention studies." *American Journal of Clinical Nutrition* 78(3 Suppl): 593S–609S.

Su, S.J. et al. 2005. "The novel targets for anti-angiogenesis of genistein on human cancer cells." *Biochemical Pharmacology* 69(2): 307–18.

**Superfruits**

Amagase, H. et al. 2009. "*Lycium barbarum* (goji) juice improves in vivo antioxidant biomarkers in serum of healthy adults." *Nutrition Research* 29(1): 19–25.

Aviram, M. et al. 2000. "Pomegranate juice consumption reduces oxidative stress, atherogenic modifications to LDL, and platelet aggregation; studies in humans and atherosclerotic apolipoprotein E-deficient mice." *American Journal of Clinical Nutrition* 71(5): 1062–76.

Aviram, M. 2002. "Pomegranate juice as a major source for polyphenolic flavonoids and it is most potent antioxidant against LDL oxidation and atherosclerosis." *Proceedings of the 11th Biennial Meeting of the Society for Free Radical Research International* 523–28.

Beecher, G.R. 1999. "Phytonutrients' role in metabolism: effects on resistance to degenerative processes." *Nutrition Review* 57(9): S3–6.

Burke, D.S. et al. 2005. "*Momordica cochinchinensis, Rosa roxburghii*, wolfberry, and sea buckthorn: highly nutritional fruits supported by tradition and science." *Current Topics in Nutraceutical Research* 3(4): 259–66.

Cao, G.W. et al. 1994, "Observation of the effects of LAK/IL–2 therapy combined with *Lycium barbarum* polysaccharides in the treatment of 75 cancer patients." *Chunghua Chung Liu Tsa Chih* 16(6): 428–31.

Cheng, C.Y. et al. 2005. "Fasting plasma zeaxanthin response to *Fructus barbarum* L. (wolfberry; Kei Tze) in a food-based human supplementation trial." *British Journal of Nutrition* 93(1): 123–30.

Del Pozo-Insfram, D. et al. 2006. "Açaí (*Euterpe oleracea* Mart.) polyphenolics in their glycoside and aglycone forms induce apoptosis of HL-60 leukemia cells." *Journal of Agriculture and Food Chemistry.* 54(4): 1222–29.

Feeney, M.J. 2004. "Fruits and the prevention of lifestyle-related diseases." *Clinical Experiments in Pharmacology and Physiology* 31(2): S11–3.

Gan, L. et al. 2003. "A polysaccharide-protein complex from *Lycium barbarum* upregulates cytokine expression in human peripheral blood mononuclear cells." *European Journal of Pharmacology* 471(3): 217–22.

He, J. et al. 1993. "Hepatoprotective effects from *Lycium barbarum* fruit in a mouse experiment." *China Pharmacology and Toxicology* 7(4): 293.

Ho, C.K. et al. 2002. "Garcinone E, a xanthone derivative, has potent cytotoxic effect against hepatocellular carcinoma cell lines." *Planta Medica* 68(11): 975–79.

Iinuma, M. et al. 1996. "Antibacterial activity of xanthones from guttiferaeous plants against methicillin-resistant *Staphylococcus aureus*." *Journal of Pharmacy & Pharmacology* 48(8): 861–65.

Jiang, D.J. et al. 2004. "Pharmacological effects of xanthones as cardiovascular protective agents." *Cardiovascular Drug Reviews* 22(2): 91–102.

Kiefer I., et al. 2004. "Supplementation with mixed fruit and vegetable juice concentrates increased serum antioxidants and folate in healthy adults." *Journal of the American College of Nutrition* 23(3): 205–11.

Matsumoto, K. et al. 2004. "Preferential target is mitochondria in α-mangostin-induced apoptosis in human leukemia HL60 cells." *Bioorganic & Medicinal Chemistry* 12(22): 5799–806.

Pantuck, A.J. et al. 2006. "Phase II study of pomegranate juice for men with rising prostate-specific antigen following surgery or radiation for prostate cancer." *Clinical Cancer Research* 12(13): 4018–26.

Rosenblat, M. et al. 2006. "Anti-oxidative effects of pomegranate juice (PJ) consumption by diabetic patients on serum and on macrophages." *Atherosclerosis* 187(2): 363–71.

Suksamrarn, S. et al. 2003. "Antimycobacterial activity of prenylated xanthones from the fruits of *Garcinia mangostana*." *Chemical & Pharmaceutical Bulletin* (Tokyo) 51(7): 857–59.

Sumner, M.D. et al. 2005. "Effects of pomegranate juice consumption on myocardial perfusion in patients with coronary heart disease." *American Journal of Cardiology* 96(6): 810–14.

Weecharangsan, W. et al. 2006. "Antioxidative and neuroprotective activities of extracts from the fruit hull of mangosteen (*Garcinia mangostana* Linn.)" *Medical Principles and Practice* 15(4): 281–87.

Williams, P. et al. 1995. "Mangostin inhibits the oxidative modification of human low density lipoprotein." *Free Radical Research* 23(2): 175–84.

**Turmeric**

Arafa, H.M. 2005. "Curcumin attenuates diet-induced hypercholesterolemia in rats." *Medical Science Monitor* 11(7): BR228–34.

Bapu, P.S. and K. Srinivasan. 1995. "Influence of dietary curcumin and cholesterol on the progression of experimentally induced diabetes in albino rat." *Molecular & Cellular Biochemistry* 152(1): 13–21.

Bundy, R. et al. 2004. "Turmeric may improve irritable bowel syndrome symptomology in otherwise healthy adults: a pilot study." *Journal of Alternative & Complementary Medicine* 10(6): 1015–18.

Funk, J.L. et al. 2006. "Turmeric extracts containing curcuminoids prevent experimental rheumatoid arthritis." *Journal of Natural Products* 69(3): 351–55.

Garcea, G. et al. "Consumption of the putative chemopreventive agent curcumin by cancer patients: assessment of curcumin levels in the colorectum and their pharmacodynamic consequences." *Cancer Epidemiology, Biomarkers & Prevention* 14(1) 120–25.

Kaur, C. and H.C. Kapoor. 2002. "Anti-oxidant activity and total phenolic content of some Asian vegetables." *International Journal of Food Science & Technology* 37(2): 153–61.

Kowluru, R.A. and M. Kanwar, 2007. "Effects of curcumin on retinal oxidative stress and inflammation in diabetes." *Nutrition & Metabolism* 4(Apr 16): 8.

Lim, G.P. et al. 2001. "The curry spice curcumin reduces oxidative damage and amyloid pathology in an Alzheimer transgenic mouse." *Journal of Neuroscience* 21(21): 8370–77.

Nagabhushan, M. and S.V. Bhide. 1992. "Curcumin as an inhibitor of cancer." *Journal of the American College of Nutrition* 11(2): 192–98.

Polasa, K. et al. 1992. "Effect of turmeric on urinary mutagens in smokers." *Mutagenesis* 7(2): 107–09.

Prucksunand, C. et al. 2001. "Phase II clinical trial on effect of the long turmeric (Curcuma longa Linn) on healing of peptic ulcer. *Southeast Asian Journal of Tropical Medicine & Public Health* 32(1): 208–15.

Salh, B. et al. 2003. "Curcumin attenuates DNB-induced murine colitis." *American Journal of Physiology. Gastrointestinal & Liver Physiology* 285(1): G235–43.

Seo, K.I. et al. 2008. "Effect of curcumin supplementation on blood glucose, plasma insulin, and glucose homeostasis related enzyme activities in diabetic db/db mice." *Molecular Nutrition & Food Research* 52(9): 995–1004.

Soni, K.B. and R. Kuttan. 1992. "Effect of oral curcumin administration on serum peroxides and cholesterol levels in human volunteers." *Indian Journal of Physiology and Pharmacology* 36(4): 273–75.

Suresh Babu, P. and K. Srinivasan. 1998. "Amelioration of renal lesions associated with diabetes by dietary curcumin in streptozotocin diabetic rats." *Molecular & Cellular Biochemistry* 181(1–2): 87–96.

Ukil, A. et al. 2003. "Curcumin, the major component of food flavour turmeric, reduces mucosal injury in trinitrobenzene sulphonic acid-induced colitis." *British Journal of Pharmacology* 139(2): 209–18.

Weil, A. "3 reasons to eat turmeric." http://www.drweil.com/drw/u/ART03001/Three-Reasons-to-Eat-Turmeric.html.

Wexler, B. 2008. *Turmeric: Spices of Life*. Salt Lake City, UT: Woodland.

**Vitamin C**

Carr, A.C. and B. Frei. 1999. "Toward a new recommended dietary allowance for vitamin C based on antioxidant and health effects in humans." *American Journal of Clinical Nutrition* 69(6): 1086–107.

Duffy, S.J. et al. 1999. "Treatment of hypertension with ascorbic acid." *Lancet* 354(9195): 2048–49.

Enstrom, J.E. et al. 1992. "Vitamin C intake and mortality among a sample of the United States population." *Epidemiology* 3(3): 194–202.

Feiz, H.R. and S. Mobarhan. 2002. "Does vitamin C intake slow the progression of gastric cancer in Heliobacter pylori–infected populations?" *Nutrition Reviews* 60(1): 34–36.

Gokce, N. et al. 1999. "Long-term ascorbic acid administration reverses endothelial vasomotor dysfunction in patients with coronary artery disease." *Circulation* 99(25): 3234–40.

Jacques, P.F. 1999. "The potential preventive effects of vitamins for cataract and age-related macular degeneration." *International Journal for Vitamin and Nutrition Research* 69(3): 198–205.

Knekt, P. et al. 2004. "Antioxidant vitamins and coronary heart disease risk: a pooled analysis of 9 cohorts." *American Journal of Clinical Nutrition* 80(6): 1508–20.

Linus Pauling Institute. 2006. "Vitamin C and the common cold." *LPI Research Newsletter.* http://lpi.oregonstate.edu/ss06/cold.html.

Osganian, S.K. et al. 2003. "Vitamin C and risk of coronary heart disease in women." *Journal of the American College of Cardiology* 42(2): 246–52.

Padayatty, S.J. et al. 2003. "Vitamin C as an antioxidant: evaluation of its role in disease prevention." *Journal of the American College of Nutrition* 22(1): 18–35.

Steinmetz, K.A. and J.D. Potter. 1996. "Vegetables, fruit, and cancer prevention: a review." *Journal of the American Dietetic Association* 96(10): 1027–39.

Yokoyama, T. et al. 2000. "Serum vitamin C concentration was inversely associated with subsequent 20-year incidence of stroke in a Japanese rural community. The Shibata Study." *Stroke* 31(10): 2287–94.

**Vitamin D**

Deluca, H.F. and M.T. Cantorna. 2001. "Vitamin D: its role and uses in immunology." *FASEB Journal* 15(14): 2579–85.

Evatt, M.L. et al. 2008. "Prevalence of vitamin D insufficiency in patients with Parkinson disease and Alzheimer disease." *Archives of Neurology* 65(10): 1348–52.

Feskanich, D. et al. 2003. "Calcium, vitamin D, milk consumption, and hip fractures: a prospective study among postmenopausal women." *American Journal of Clinical Nutrition* 77(2): 504–11.

Giovannucci, E. et al. 2008. "25-hydroxyvitamin D and risk of myocardial infarction in men: a prospective study." *Archives of Internal Medicine* 168(11): 1174–80.

Holick, M.F. 2003. "Vitamin D: a millennium perspective." *Journal of Cellular Biochemistry* 88(2): 296–307.

Hyppönen, E. et al. 2001. "Intake of vitamin D and risk of type 1 diabetes: a birth-cohort study." *Lancet* 358(9292): 1500–03.

Lappe, J.M. et al. 2007. "Vitamin D and calcium supplementation reduces cancer risk: results of a randomized trial." *American Journal of Clinical Nutrition* 85(6): 1586–91.

Lips, P. et al. 2006. "The prevalence of vitamin D inadequacy amongst women with osteoporosis: an international epidemiological investigation." *Journal of Internal Medicine* 260(3): 245–54.

Melamed, M.L. et al. 2008. "25-hydroxyvitamin D levels and the risk of mortality in the general population." *Archives of Internal Medicine* 168(15): 1629–37.

Merlino, L.A. et al. 2004. "Vitamin D intake is inversely associated with rheumatoid arthritis: results from the Iowa Women's Health Study." *Arthritis and Rheumatism* 50(1): 72–77.

Munger, K.L. et al. 2006. "Serum 25-hydroxyvitamin D levels and risk of multiple sclerosis." *JAMA* 296(23): 2832–38.

Pilz, S. et al. 2008. "Low vitamin D levels predict stroke in patients referred to coronary angiography." *Stroke* 39(9): 2611–13.

Standing Committee on the Scientific Evaluation of Dietary Reference Intakes. 1997. *DRI Dietary Reference Intakes for Calcium, Phosphorus, Magnesium, Vitamin D, and Fluoride.* Washington, DC: National Academy Press.

Sutton, A.L. and P.N. MacDonald. 2003. "Vitamin D: more than a 'bone-a-fide' hormone." *Molecular Endocrinology* 17(5): 777–91.

Wagner, et a;. 2008. "Prevention of rickets and vitamin D deficiency in infants, children, and adolescents." *Pediatrics* 122(5): 1142–52.

Wang, T.J. 2008. "Vitamin D deficiency and risk of cardiovascular disease." *Circulation* 117(4): 503–11.

Zittermann, A. 2003. "Vitamin D in preventive medicine: are we ignoring the evidence?" *British Journal of Nutrition* 89(5): 552–72.

### Vitamin K

Booth, S.L. et al. 1995. "Assessment of dietary phylloquinone intake and vitamin K status in postmenopausal women." *European Journal of Clinical Nutrition* 49(11):832–41.

Booth, S.L. and J.W. Suttie. 1998. "Dietary intake and adequacy of vitamin K." *Journal of Nutrition* 128(5): 785–88.

Braam, L.A. et al. 2003. "Vitamin K1 supplementation retards bone loss in postmenopausal women between 50 and 60 years of age." *Calcified Tissue International* 73(1): 21–26.

Geleijnse, J.M. et al. 2004. "Beyond deficiency: potential benefits of increased intakes of vitamin K for bone and vascular health." *European Journal of Nutrition* 43(6): 325–35.

Hodges, S.J. et al. 1991. "Depressed levels of circulating menaquinones in patients with osteoporotic fractures of the spine and femoral neck." *Bone* 12(6): 387–89.

Iwamoto, I. et al. 1999. "A longitudinal study of the effect of vitamin K2 on bone mineral density in postmenopausal women: a comparative study with vitamin D3 and estrogen-progestin therapy." *Maturitas* 31(2): 161–64.

Jie, K.S. et al. 1995. "Vitamin K intake and osteocalcin levels in women with and without aortic atherosclerosis: a population-based study." *Atherosclerosis* 116(1): 117–23.

Kawashima, H. et al. 1997. "Effects of vitamin K2 (menatetrenone) on atherosclerosis and blood coagulation in hypercholesterolemic rabbits." *Japanese Journal of Pharmacology* 75(2): 135–43.

Meunier, P.J. 1999. "Calcium, vitamin D, and vitamin K in the prevention of fractures due to osteoporosis." *Osteoporosis International* 9(Suppl 2): S48–52.

Weber, P. 2001. "Vitamin K and bone health." *Nutrition* 17(10): 880–87.

# Index